CW00446639

Psychoneuroimmunology

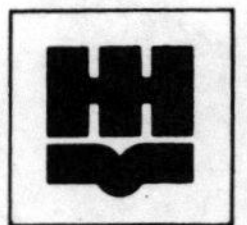

Psychoneuro-immunology

Interactions between Brain, Nervous System, Behavior, Endocrine and Immune System

Edited by
Hans-Joachim Schmoll
Uwe Tewes
Medical University
Hannover, F.R.G.
Nicholas P. Plotnikoff
University of Illinois
Chicago, U.S.A.

Hogrefe & Huber Publishers
Lewiston, NY · Toronto · Bern · Göttingen

Library of Congress Cataloging-in-Publication Data

Psychoimmunology : interactions between brain, nervous system, behavior, endocrine, and immune system / edited by Hans-Joachim Schmoll, Uwe Tewes, Nicholas P. Plotnikoff.
Based on an international symposium which took place in Sept. 1989 in Hannover, Germany.
Includes bibliographical references and index.
ISBN 0-88937-067-2. — ISBN 3-456-82086-0
1. Psychoneuroimmunology—Congresses. I. Schmoll, H.-J. (Hans-Joachim). II. Tewes, Uwe. III. Plotnikoff, Nicholas P.
[DNLM: 1. Behavior—congresses. 2. Brain—immunology—congresses. 3. Endocrine Glands—immunology—congresses. 4. Immune System—physiology—congresses. WL 103 P97353 1989]
QP356.47.P78 1991
616.07′9′019-dc20
DNLM/DLC
for Library of Congress 91-35385 CIP

Canadian Cataloguing in Publication Data

Main entry under title:
Psychoneuroimmunology

Papers presented at an international symposium held Sept. 1989 in Hannover, Germany.
Includes bibliographical references and index.
ISBN 0-88937-067-2

1. Psychoneuroimmunology—Congresses. I. Schmoll, Hans-Joachim. II. Tewes, Uwe. III. Plotnikoff, Nicholas P.

QP356.47.P78 1992 616.07′9 C91-095723-1

P. O. Box 51
Lewiston, NY 14092

12–14 Bruce Park Ave.
Toronto, Ontario M4P 2S3

ISBN 0-88937-067-2
ISBN 3-456-82086-0
Hogrefe & Huber Publishers
Lewiston, NY · Toronto · Bern · Göttingen

Printed in Germany on acid-free paper

Preface

Even until a few years ago the immune system had been described to be an autonomous system functioning independently from other biological and psychological systems of regulator processes. With our increasing understanding of how the immunesystem functions, it is now clear that this extraordinarily complex system is closely interlinked with other systems of the organism, particularly the endocrine and the nervous systems. Since animal experiments indicated that immunological reactions can be conditioned, the classical theory of psychogenesis of somatic diseases was reformulated. Now the question is how psychological factors possibly modulate the function of the immune system via neurohormones.

Thus, since the early Eighties, a cooperative approach in research gained increasing importance, and was frequently and somewhat simply called "psychoneuroimmunology" in the literature. Under this collective heading immunologists, endocrinologists, neurologists, neurophysiologists, pharmacologists, psychologists, oncologists, and psychiatrists are cooperating in studying the interrelations between psychological, neurological, endocrinological, and immunological processes.

This volume is intended to repeat, in a relativly paradigmatic fashion, on interdisciplinary research approaches in this field. As to the background of this publication, we would like to mention, that two of the editors have already organized in October 1988 a workshop at the Medical University of Hannover entitled "Psychoneuroimmunology in Oncology". When, in December 1988, the Volkswagen Foundation established a new main research area named "Neuroimmunologie, Verhalten und Befinden", we applied to fund an International Symposium on the topic which the the title of this book reflects. This took place in September 1989 in Hannover. The papers presented were critically reviewed by the editors, who finally decided to present here those contributions which provided a good insight into the breadth scope of studies in this new field of research. The results presented cover primarily the areas of Immunology, Neurobiology, Endocrinology, Cell Biology, and Pharmacology, as well as findings in Psychology, Psychosomatics and Psychiatry.

H.-J. Schmoll U. Tewes N. Plotnikoff

Contents

Part I

Brain, Behavior, Nervous System, and Immunity

Chapter 1

Introduction: Psychoneuroimmunology - an Overview

Hugo O. Besedowsky
Division of Neurobiology
University Hospital, Basel

The immune system is built up of an enormous variety of interacting cells and molecules. The amount of information that it can process and the different responses that it can generate probably make the immune system the most complex body system after the CNS. Furthermore, since under natural conditions changes in the activity of the immune system are often linked to disease, it operates at the diffuse border between physiological and pathophysiological processes. Therefore, the integration of immune mechanisms with mechanisms under brain control is necessarily complex. So many variables play or can potentially play a role in immune-CNS communication that the only conceivable basis for such a communication is a network of immune-neuro-endocrine interactions.

In my view, the biological implications of such a network are as follows:

I The immune system behaves as a receptor-sensorial organ which informs central neuro-endocrine structures about ongoing immune responses.

II Immune-neuroendocrine circuits contribute to the regulation of the immune response.

III The immune system, through its capacity to produce hormone-like substances, also participates in the control of host neuro-endocrine and metabolic adjustments, e.g., metabolic adjustments during infective, inflammatory and neoplastic processes.

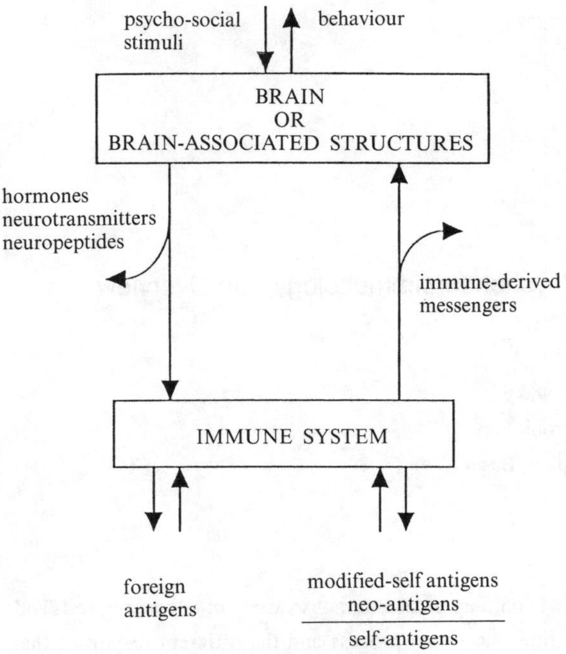

Fig. 1: The Immune Neuro-Endocrine Network

How is the immune-neuro-endocrine network organized? A realistic scheme of such a network would consist of an enormous number of interconnected arrows (and question marks!) since each component of this network (the immune system, the CNS, the peripheral neuro-endocrine and immunohormonal circuits) is itself a system based on interconnected elements. Thus, for reasons of clarity, an oversimplified diagram is shown in Fig. 1. The ascending arrow from the immune system to the CNS represents the receptor/sensorial component, and the descending arrow the regulatory component of the network. From these ascending and descending pathways, two shorter arrows branch out symbolizing effects that the operation of the immune-neuro-endocrine network will exert on general host homeostasis.

The intrusion of foreign antigens represents a disturbance of the homeostasis. On the other hand, self antigens present on cell membranes and in body fluids can be considered as biological markers of cell and tissue constancy and integrity. Modified self-antigens and neo-antigens represent alterations in the cellular constituents of the body. Therefore, the immune system, due to its capacity to discriminate self from non-self, can perceive an internal image of body constituents and react to particular distortions of this image. However, there is now evidence that the immune system not only responds to antigens but also conveys messages to central structures. In fact, some lympho-monokines, complement fractions, antibodies, classical neurotransmitters such as histamine and serotonin and even immune-derived peptide hormones can affect neuro-endocrine structures. Depending on the type of antigenic stimulus, multiple possible combinations of products derived from subsets of lymphoid and accessory cells would occur. Viewed thus, one can conceive of a code based on combinations of soluble messengers which could inform the central nervous system about the type of immune response in operation. Also, information about the site of an ongoing immune response could be transmitted by stimulation of autonomic and sensorial nerve fibers innervating "strategically" located lymphoid organs or tissues affected by infective or inflammatory processes. The existence of an afferent pathway from the immune system to the CNS implies, as we have suggested, that the immune system is a receptor/sensorial organ.

After receiving signals from the immune system, the brain or brain-controlled structures may or may not respond by emitting regulatory signals. If brain intervention does occur, the regulatory outcome will be the result of both external neuro-endocrine signals acting at specific receptors on immunological cells and of autoregulatory immunological signals. In fact, increasing evidence showing the capacity of certain hormones, neurotransmitters and neuropeptides to affect regulatory mechanisms intrinsic to the immune system is available. This view of immunoregulation provides a broader framework which contrasts with the concept of a self-contained, self-monitored immune system.

A circuitry involving immunological cell products and neuro-endocrine agents will necessarily have consequences for the whole organism and will affect general homeostasis (Fig. 1, branching out arrows). Homeostatic mechanisms under basal conditions may differ qualitatively or quantitatively from those which operate during pathological states involving the immune system. In fact, there is evidence that the set points for the regulation of essential variables are adjusted at different levels during the course of these states. Immunohormones and/or immunotransmitters may contribute to the integration of these adjustments either directly or through their effects on neuro-endocrine mechanisms. When these adjustments are appropriate, they would be beneficial for the host; otherwise, they may aggravate the course of the disease.

This view of immune-neuro-endocrine interactions as a network allows us to assume that the degree of activity of the network can be changed by stimuli acting at or generated from any of its components, e.g. antigens at the level of the immune system, psycho-social stimuli at the level of the CNS. This will have consequences for both immune responses and behaviour. It can also be assumed that the tonic functioning of the network would maintain the connectivity between the various components, thus keeping them informed about their respective functional states. This concept would also allow a more integrative interpretation of certain findings, e.g. "stress conditions and certain psychiatric diseases influence the immune system" could be thought of as "during stress conditions or certain psychiatric diseases, the degree of interactions with the network is altered". Behavioral conditioning of the immune response can also be interpreted as a process that affects certain connections of a constantly operating network of brain-immune interactions. Furthermore, a progressive and cumulative deterioration of the connectivity within the network may be an important component of aging. There are so many levels at which immune processes could be controlled that monocausal interpretations of its functioning are not realistic. It is necessary to take into account the convergence of signals coming from within or outside the immune system. This integrative view often makes the boundaries between disciplines very diffuse. Hormones, neurotransmitters, neuropeptides and lympho-monokines constantly exchange roles. Neuro-endocrine agents can act as messengers within the immune system and immunological cell products can participate in the control of CNS functions. Furthermore, immunological processes are metabolically very demanding and we now know that immune cell products can also affect general metabolism. A network of interactions that involves distinct and essential body agencies is, as pointed out at the beginning, necessarily complex. However, the control of complex biological networks is in the domain of physiology. Thus, as reflected by the different topics discussed during this symposium, we may be beginning to understand the physiology of the immune system within an integrated organism. We should also be aware that we have to face the eternal dilemma of physiology: one can isolate structures but not functions, and one can purify messengers but not signals.

Chapter 2

The Relation between Social Rank and Chronic Inflammatory Responses,on Different Genetic Backgrounds: Experimental Studies in Inbred Rats

Klaus Gärtner
Karl A. Mensing
Reinhard Velleuer

Central Animal Laboratories
Hannover Medical University

The following paper intends to show psychoimmune modulations as mechanisms supporting natural selection. The paper may help to answer the question: What is the biological advantage in the interaction between behaviour, and the endocrine and immune system, that was developed in mammals including man. The question was studied in experiments by comparing relative Darwin fitness (social rank), with susceptibility to Mycoplasma arthritidis.

Methods

Fig. 1 summarizes the methods, and the first results of our studies on the relation between social rank and the clinical course of an experimental infection with Mycoplasma arthritidis in male inbred rats, which are described in detail elsewhere (Gärtner et al., 1989; Velleuer, 1986; Mensing, 1987).

Estimation of social rank. From the different types of social hierarchies in groups of rats (territorial, food competition and so on) we estimated the type, which is best linked with the relative Darwinian fitness of each male. Healthy male rats, caged in groups of four, were confronted with one estric female for 100 min at 10 days. The frequencies of copulatory patterns of each male were counted under such competitive conditions. Frequently, there were one or two males in each cage, which were performing significantly more ejaculations than the others. From other experiments (Gärtner et al., 1986, 1989), we know that these rats may sire perhaps75 % of the next generation. Their Darwinian fitness is the highest. We call such rats "A-males". Other males, that we call "O-males", show few copulatory performances and sire only 5 %. B-males are of intermediate sexual activity and may sire about 20 %.

Experimental infection with M. arthritidis. After having estimated the social rank of the healthy animals in this way, we intravenously injected the four males Mycoplasma arthritidis germs (strain ISR 1 (Kirchhoff et al. ,1983),108 colony forming units) at day 0. They were examined afterwards, every two or four days, over a period of 110 days. Twenty clinical and laboratory characteristics were recorded in each of the 156 animals. The graphs (Fig. 1) summarize the results by showing the course of the disease using two guide-line characteristics: (1) the reduction of body weight, and (2) the degree of polyarthritis. Both characteristics were investigated with respect to time, from day 0 to day 110. In order to quantitatively compare the severity of disease between the individuals, the area bound by the graph was calculated for each animal and each clinical parameter, as shown by the hatching in Fig. 1, below.

Results

Strain differences. The experiments were done using males of three different inbred strains: DA/Ztm, AS/Ztm, LEW/Ztm. The Animals are bred in our own breeding colony, and are barrier-derived SPF-animals. Cage mates are always of the same age. Remembering that all males of an inbred strain are genotypically identical we can conclude that any differences between strains will therefore represent genotypic variability. The columns show the effects on the polyarthritis score during the chronic period after infection between day 40 and day110. More genetic results are described by Gärtner et al. (1989) and Binder et al. (1990) The results demonstrate the well known influence of different genotypes on the severity of this disease. Animals from the DA strain showed relatively low polyarthritis scores when compared with animals of the inbred strains AS and LEW. Heritability in a broader sense was calculated at about 0.6 - 0.8, the same as we estimated in other series between 23 inbred strains. (Binder et al., 1990). Both the body weight reduction and also the other clinical characteristics, estimated

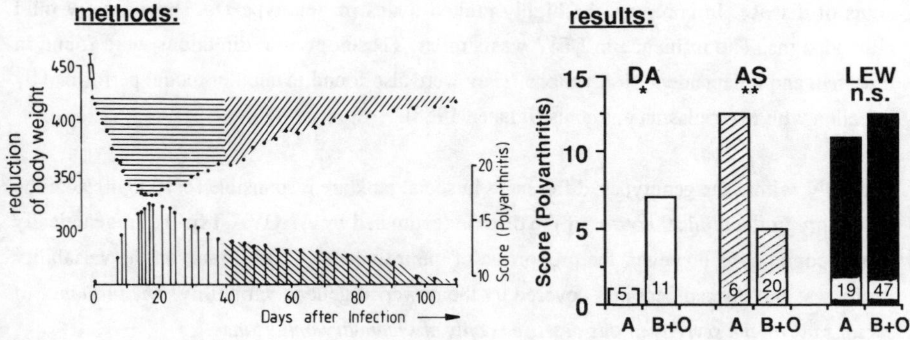

Fig. 1: left (Methods): Estimation of Relative Darwin Fitness, Infection, Calculation of Body Weight Reduction and Polyarthritis Score for each Male Rat over Time
right (Results): Influence of Relative Darwin Fitness (Social Ranks A, B, O) on the Susceptibility to M. Arthritis in Inbred Strains (DA/Ztm, AS/Ztm, LEW/Ztm) of Adult Male Rats

during either the acute or chronic period, are similarly influenced by genetic diversities. From these results we drew the general conclusion: genetic differences are the most powerful component influencing the variability of this disease.

Influence of social rank. We observed the influence of social rank within each inbred strain. Within each inbred strain the influences of rank are compared between the A-ranked rats and the others. Each column represents animals of similar social rank: the left columns represent males with high copulatory efficiency, called A-males. The right columns represent animals of intermediate (B) and little efficient animals (O). These two types are combined due to statistical reasons. Remember that any differences within inbred strains are caused solely by behavioural differences, and not by the interactions of genotype and psychotype, as all males of an inbred strain are isogenic.

Firstly, I want to underline the most important information of my paper: the finding that the *influence of rank has a vice-versa direction between the genotypes*. This is very obvious between DA and AS. The highly ranked A-males of genotype AS showed the strongest clinical signs of disease. In contrary, the highly ranked males of genotype DA showed very mild clinical signs. The influence in LEW was similar. These opposite directions were found in repeated, and independent observations. They were also found in another model performed by infection with Mycoplasma pulmonis (Iglauer, 1988).

Secondly, within the genotypes, differences in social rank are responsible for10 to 40 % of the variability in the clinical course of the disease (estimated by ANOVA Typ II). In genetically mixed populations however, the proportion of the influence of social rank on the variability decreases, and instead becomes covered by the powerful genetic variability. *The influence of social rank on the severity of this desease is only of secundary importance.*

The contrary influence of social rank on the severity of the illness in different genotypes helps to understand the well known difficulties in estimating correlations between social rank and chronic inflammation under field conditions and in human populations. In natural populations these vice-versa reacting genotypes are mixed. This may prevent the discovery of such correlations, such as those which we were able to show in the different models of inbred animals.

Estimation of the somatic, endocrine and immunological pathways which are responsible for the correlation between social rank and the severity of chronic inflammation.The scheme in Fig. 2 summarizes some of the pathways which are in discussion.In the model of M. arthritidis, we examined the influence of social rank only at the six marked points, which we took as markers for the endocrine general adaptative syndrome, and the catecholaminergic emergency reaction. From the results, both the influence of social rank on the correlation between local inflammation (as measured by the polyarthritis score) as well as on the disposal of specific antibodies in the plasma, is summarized in Fig. 2.

Immune suppression by social rank. Fig. 3 summarizes the results in animals of the strain LEW. The ordinate shows the polyarthritis- scores which were integrated over day 1 - 39 of the disease in the animals. The abscissa shows the specific antibodies of the plasma integrated over the same period. Stars show the values from A-males which perform a linear regression ($p < 0.01$). We calculated the shown regression line from the A-males. Fig. 3 shows that the results of animals low in rank (B and O) are frequently above this regression line. 41 lower-ranked males were above this regression line and only 12 below the line. The A-males showed the expected equilibrated distribution. The difference is statistically significant ($p < 0.01$) (see Tab. in Fig. 3, right). In other words, in classes of the same degree of local inflammation (shown by the interrupted horizontal lines), the lower ranked animals have a

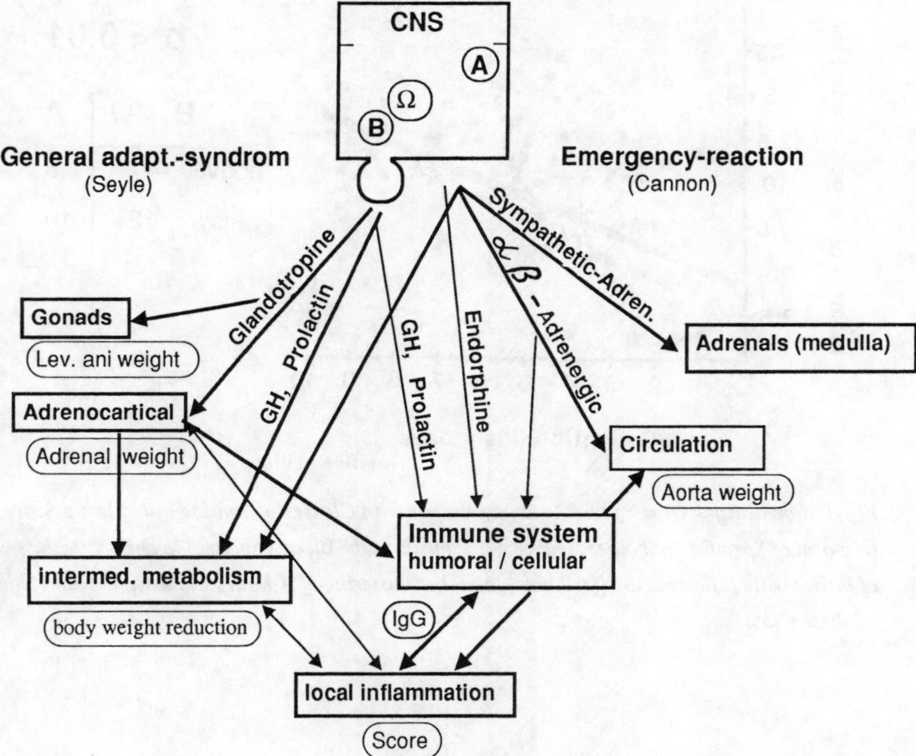

Fig. 2: PathwaysConnecting Central Nervous System, Endocrine Sytem, and Inflammatory Process.

depressed and probably inapprop-priated humoral immune response in comparison to the A-males. We therefore suppose that a suppressed disposal of specific antibodies in the plasma and in the inflammated tissue in the low ranked animals of strain LEW are caused by the specific psychosocial conditions and also by the well known. desequilibration of their endocrine system, an issue which has been described by v. Holst et.al. (1983) for tree shrews, and also by Gärtner et al. (1980) for rats of our strains.

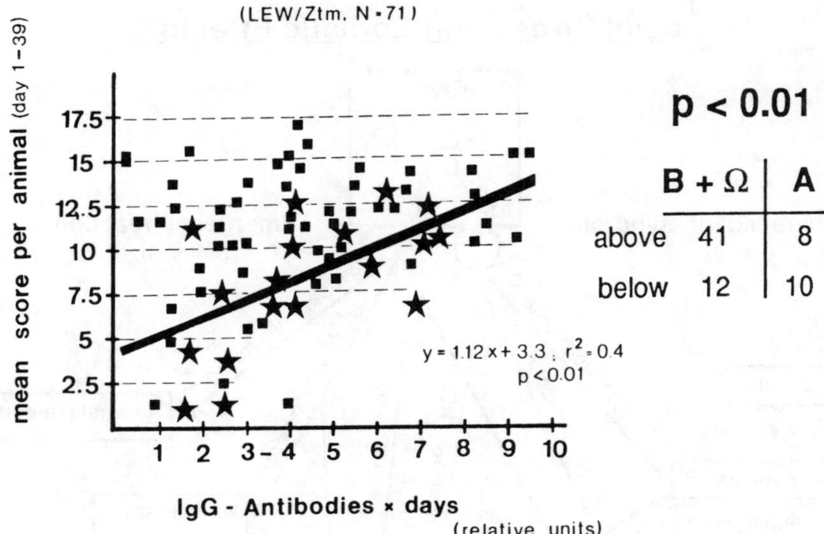

*Fig. 3: Social Rank (A = *) and Antibody Response in Classes of Similar Polyathritis-Score. Disposal of Specific Antibodies Against M. Arthritis in the Blood (Abcisse) in Different Classes of Polyathritic Inflammation (Ordinate), and the Clustering of A-Males at the Right Hand Side od these Classes.*

Similar results were also seen in the strain DA. But strain AS with the severily diseased A-males is in contrary to the conditions in the strains DA and LEW: the most severe diseased A-males are in the upper left corner of a similar triangle of the distribution (for details see Gärtner et al., 1989). From recent results with experimental infections caused by Mycoplasma pulmonis we know that not only B-cell functions but also the T-cells and the bronchial associated lymphatic tissue (BALT) are reduced (Gerdes, 1988).

Discussion

Psychoimmune modulations as mechanisms supporting natural selection.

What is the biological significance of the diverse (if you regard different genotypes) correlation between social rank and immune suppression, in general and in particular? Perhaps we are seeing here part of the mechanism which supports natural selection. This is demonstrated by Fig. 4.

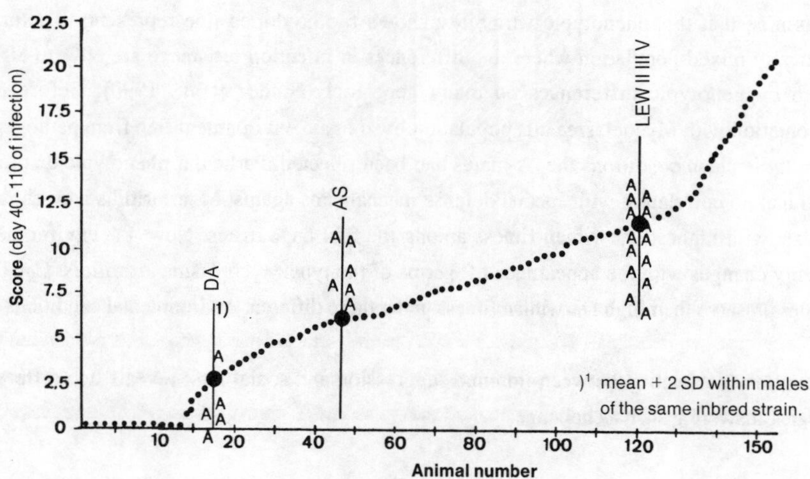

Fig. 4: Polyathritis-Score (40 - 110 Days after Infection) of 152 Male Rats Classified According to the Severity (small dots), and Derived from the inbred Strains AS/Ztm, DA/Ztm, LEW/Ztm. Strain Mean +/- 2 SD (Thin Vertical Lines) of the Inbred Strain and Position of A-Males on the Vertical Line.

They are classified according to the severity of the arthritis scores which each animal exhibits 40 - 110 days after infection. A continuous variability is shown. In15 animals the joints were not injured, 110 animals had moderate inflammations of the joints with scores from 0.1 to 12, and about 30 animals were severely ill. The dotted line represents the different courses of the disease in individuals of a genetically mixed population - similar to a natural population - with three known genotypes.

For comparison, the vertical lines represent the means and the ranges of the scores for animals of the same genotype. In these ranges, the positions of the A-males are marked. In the LEW strain the values for the A-males are below the mean value. This is shown by the fact that their individual points are all on the left hand side of the genotypic mean (represented by a large point) on the dotted line. In the AS strain, the A-males are above the mean; shown because all their individual points are on the right hand side from the genotypic mean (again represented by a large point) on the dotted line.

We assume that this phenotypic variability shown by the dotted line represents a natural, genetically mixed population where the differences in infection resistance are 60% to 80 % caused by genotypic differences on many gene loci (Binder et al., 1990). Before the confrontation with Mycoplasma this population lived in an environment free from pathogens. Under these clean conditions the A-males had been selected. Particular phenotypic qualities which had no correlation with special defense mechanisms against M. arthritidis had chosen the male with highest Darwinian fitness among the four cage mates. Now the environment suddenly changes with the appearance of germs of the type Mycoplasma arthritidis. Can the A-males preserve their high Darwinian fitness under these different environmental conditions?

The contrary correlation between immune suppression and social rank reveals two different strategies answering such a challenge:

The first strategy is shown in the AS-strain: there is a strong linkage between high rank and immune suppression. So the A-position causes a severe illness.The A-males were tested very strong. A-males may loose their rank position. Males of lower ranks, which have fallen ill less severely, will take over their rank place, as we have observed in this strain. By such a strategy, a population will quickly change to the left end of the scale shown in Fig. 4.

The very different, second strategy is shown in the strains LEW by the linkage of high social rank with higher resistance against the infection.The A-males have a bonus of resistance in comparison with their cage mates during the confrontation with Mycoplasma arthritidis. The

The very different, second strategy is shown in the strains LEW by the linkage of high social rank with higher resistance against the infection.The A-males have a bonus of resistance in comparison with their cage mates during the confrontation with Mycoplasma arthritidis. The selection of other animals, more resistant against infections but lower in social rank, is depressed. Perhaps this strategy preserves the genotypes of the A-males for other biological reasons.

Probably both strategies are present in a natural population . They may be caused by different allels of genes, which are responsible for the interaction between behaviour and the endocrine and the immune system.

References

Binder, A.K.U., Gärtner, K., Hedrich, H.J., Hermanns, W., Kirchhoff, H. & Wonigeit, K. (1990). Strain differences in the sensitivity of rats to Mycoplasma arthritidis ISR 1 infection are under multiple gene control. *Infection and Immunity 58:* 1584-1590.

Gärtner, K., Döhler, K. & Rechenberg, I. (1980). Internal selection and hormonal balance in rat population. In: Stark, E., Makara, G.B., Endröczi, E. (Eds.) *Adv Physiol Sci Vol 13, Endocrinology, Neuroendocrinology, Neuropeptides 1,* Pergamon Press.

Gärtner, K., Amelang, D., Bredereck, W. & Tessmer, Ch. (1986). Promiskuitive Kopulation bei Laboratoriumsratten. *Fertilität 2:* 224-230.

Gärtner, K., Kirchhoff, H., Mensing, K. & Velleuer, R. (1989). The influence of social rank on the susceptibility of rats to Mycoplasma arthritidis. *J Behav Med 12:* 487-502.

Gerdes, E. (1988). *Genetische und psychosoziale Einflüsse auf das pathologisch-anatomische und -histologische Bild der Murinen Respiratorischen Mykoplasmose bei Lew/Ztm- und AS/Ztm-Ratten.* Vet. med. Diss. Hannover.

Holst, D. v., Fuchs, E. & Stör, W. (1983). Physiological changes in male Tupaia belangeri under different types of social stress. In: T.M. Dembrowski, T.H. Schmidt, G. Blümchen (Eds.): *Biobehavioural bases of coronary diseases. Karger biobehavioural medicine series. Vol. 2.* Karger, Basel.

Iglauer, F. (1988). *Entwicklung eines Modelles zur Untersuchung psychosozialer und genetischer Einflüsse auf den Verlauf einer chronisch respiratorischen Erkrankung (Murine Respiratorische Mykoplasmose) bei der Ratte.* Vet. med. Diss. Hannover.

Kirchhoff, H., Heitmann, J., Ammar, A., Hermanns, W. & Schulz, L.-C. (1983). Studies of Polyarthritis Caused by Mycoplasma arthritidis in Rats. I. Detection of the Persisting Mycoplasma Antigen by the Enzyme Immune Assay (EIA) and Conventional Culture Technique. *Zentralbl Bakteriol Abt 1, Orig. A 254:* 129-138.

Mensing, K.-A. (1987). *Verlauf und Schwere einer experimentellen Infektion mit Mycoplasma arthritidis bei der Ratte und Einfluß von Psychotypen.* Vet. med. Diss. Hannover.

Velleuer, R. (1986). *Entwicklung eines Modelles zur Untersuchung genetischer und psychosozialer Einflüsse auf den Verlauf einer experimentellen Infektion mit Mycoplasma arthritidis bei der Ratte.* Vet. med. Diss. Hannover.

Chapter 3

Cerebral Lateralisation and Immunity

Pierre J. Neveu
INSERM U259 University Bordeaux II

Functional and neuroanatomical studies have demonstrated that the brain is lateralized in humans and many other animal species. There is a general agreement that the two cerebral hemispheres contribute differentially to the regulation of human behaviour (Levy, 1974). Moreover, the two hemispheres may be differently involved in psychiatric and neurological diseases (Bruder et al., 1989; Flor-Henry, 1976; Maaser and Farley, 1988). Morphological brain asymmetries have been described in humans for some time now (Habib and Galaburda, 1986), and the asymmetrical distribution of neurotransmitters found in human and rodent brains is correlated with the functional heterogeneity of the two hemispheres (Glick et al., 1979; 1982; Oke et al., 1980; Barnéoud et al., 1990a). Not only are some number of brain functions lateralized but the central nervous system modulates the activity of the immune system. One implication is that the brain may regulate immune responses in an asymmetrical manner. In the early 1980's, two different paradigms were used to demonstrate that indeed the two hemispheres modulate immune functions differently. First, left or right cortical ablations in mice had opposite effects on several immunological parameters. Left cortical lesions depressed T-lymphocyte functions whereas symmetrical right ablation had no or even enhancing effects (Renoux et al., 1983). Secondly, Geshwind and Behan (1982) described an association between left-handedness in humans and incidence of immune disorders.

Recent work, using neuroanatomical approach, has confirmed and extended the opposite effects of left and right cortical ablations on immune parameters. In mice tested six to ten weeks after ablation of the left fronto-parieto-occipital cortex (group L) mitogen-induced T-cell proliferation was decreased. After a similar lesion of the right neocortex (group R) mitogenesis was enhanced (Renoux et al., 1983; Neveu et al., 1986). Differences were statistically significant only when left hemisphere- and right hemisphere-lesioned groups were compared. Most often, however neither group differed from the unoperated control group. These modifications in T-cell proliferation have been shown to parallel interleukin-2 production (Neveu et al., 1989c). Additionaly, natural killer cell activity was impaired after left cortical ablations (Renoux et al., 1983a; Betancur et al., 1990b). Cortical lesions also modified, but only slightly and without statistical significance, mitogen-induced proliferation of B-cells (Neveu et al., 1986). Production of antibodies of the IgG isotype (T-dependent) but not IgM antibody synthesis (T-independent) was depressed after left lesions (Renoux et al., 1983). Finally, brain neocortex modulates macrophage activation (Neveu et al., 1989a). The intraperitoneal injection of Calmette-Guérin bacillus is known to induce an accumulation of activated macrophages in the peritoneum. A similar accumulation was not observed after cortical lesions, mainly to the left hemisphere. Moreover oxidative metabolism was decreased in animals of group L as compared to group R or controls. The function of non-activated resident macrophages was not affected by damaging the cortex. Likewise, IL-1 production by macrophages stimulated by LPS is depressed after left lesions but enhanced after right lesions (Qiu-Shi and Gui-Zhen, 1987). Similar asymmetrical brain neocortex modulation of T cell mitogenesis has been reported for rats (Barnéoud et al., 1988b).

Other evidence for brain asymmetrical modulation of the immune system comes from a functional approach and follows the observation of a higher incidence of immune disorders in left-handed humans (Geshwind and Behan, 1982). However, other researchers have failed to replicate those findings (Betancur et al., 1990; Cosi et al., 1988; Pennington et al., 1987; Salcedo et al., 1985), and original studies remain controversial both on theoretical and methodological grounds (Satz and Soper, 1986; Wofsy, 1984). In order to overcome the difficulties encountered in human studies, we recently initiated a research program in laboratory animals. We have demonstrated an association between asymmetrical brain function and immune responses of mice. Animals may be selected for right- or left-handedness using a paw-preference test described by Collins (1985). Left-handed, in contrast to right-handed mice may be characterized as having 1) higher mitogen-induced T lymphocyte proliferation in C3H/He females (Neveu et al., 1988b) but no in C3H/OuJIco males, 2) lower NK cell activity in C3H/OuJIco males (Betancur et al., 1991) and earlier auto-antibody production in females of the NZB strain but not in males (Neveu et al., 1989b).

The brain structures involved in neocortex-mediated immunomodulation is still under investigation. First, the respective role of each hemisphere in neocortex mediated immunomodulation remains controversial. Renoux and Bizière (1986) have postulated that the right hemicortex modulates the activity of the left, which in turn controls the immune system. According to this hypothesis, the effects of bilateral cortical ablation should be similar to those of left lesion alone. Indeed, they have shown that both bilateral lesions (two unilateral lesions performed within a time interval of 3 weeks to avoid mortality observed after one stage bilateral damage) did not modify mitogen-induced lymphoproliferation (Neveu et al., 1988a). Suppression of the asymmetrical immunoregulatory effects by bilateral cortical ablation suggested that each hemicortex may be active on the immune system in opposing fashion. The right hemisphere may increase while the left depressed T-cell functions. More recently, we have found that left, but not right, cortical ablation abolished the difference in T-lymphocyte responsiveness observed between right- and left-handed mice (Neveu et al., 1991). These results suggest that only the left hemisphere may be involved in the association between handedness and immunity. Furthermore, each hemicortex appears to be heterogenous in relation to its immunoregulatory functions. The consequences of unilateral lesions restricted to the parieto-occipital areas are different from those observed after lesions involving all of the fronto-parieto-occipital cortex (Barnéoud et al., 1987; Neveu, 1988). That modulation of immunological parameters may be different as a function of size of the lesion suggests that each hemisphere may contain both activating and suppressing areas which may interact both within and between hemispheres.

Neurochemical changes induced by unilateral ablation of the cortex may provide information on the subcortical structures involved in brain immunomodulation (Barnéoud et al, 1990b). Unilateral cortical ablation induced profound and widespread changes 14 days after surgery in the contralateral cortex as well as in subcortical regions of both sides. Lesions of the left neocortex appeared mainly to affect the activity of the serotoninergic inputs to the right neocortex, whereas ablations of the right cortex influenced the activity of the catecholaminergic inputs to the left. Sixty days after surgery, modifications in monoamine levels were observed only in the ipsilateral, but not contralateral subcortical regions. The only exception was that dopamine turnover in the tuberoinfundibular system remained lowered in both hemispheres after either right or left cortical ablations. On the other hand, left and right-handed subpopulations of mice which exhibit different reactivity of lymphocytes differ according to asymmetrical distributions of cortical and bulbospinal noradrenaline content as well as dopamine turnover, in the tuberoinfundibular system (Barnéoud et al., 1990a). The only relations between lesion and paw-preference were observed for dopamine and DOPAC concentrations in the anterior hypothalamus when studying chronic changes, 60 days after cortical lesions (Barnéoud et al., 1990a). Differences in dopamine levels between the right and left hemispheres observed in left-handed mice were abolished after cortical lesions. An asymmetry in the opposite direction was found for DOPAC levels in left-handed sham operated animals. This asymmetry persisted after a right lesion but not after a left one (Barnéoud et al., 1991). It may be suggested that the left neocortex is involved in neuroimmunomodulation through the dopaminergic tuberoinfundibular system. In agreement with this hypothesis, dopamine from the tuberoinfundibular region is known to inhibit prolactine production which is known to be a potent immunomodulator (Bernton, 1989; Cross and Roszman, 1989). Experimental verification of the hypothesis will require that the role of hypothalamic neurons be assessed more directly.

Other central dopaminergic structures appear to be involved in asymmetrical brain immunomodulation. We have recently shown that 4 and 6 weeks after left or right lesions of substantia nigra, spleen lymphocyte mitogenesis was slightly depressed or enhanced respectively as compared to sham-operated controls. Differences appeared with comparisons of left and right lesioned groups. However, natural killer cell activity was unaffected by unilateral lesions of substantia nigra (Neveu et al., submitted). Furthermore, 14 days after these unilateral lesions, alterations of lymphocytes mitogenesis were quite similar to those previously observed after unilateral cortex ablations (Barnéoud et al., 1988a). On the other hand, the contribution of the substantia nigra is not clear for difference in immune reactivity between left and right-handed mice which we reported earlier. In previous unpublished work, we failed to find asymmetrical distribution of dopamine in the striatum, and dopamine metabolism in both striata was similar for right- or left-handed animals. Nevertheless, the skilled use of one forelimb, has been shown to be related to dopamine in the striatum (Wishaw et al., 1986).

Among the subcortical structures known to send projections to the neocortex, the nucleus basalis magnocellularis provides the major source of cortical cholinergic innervation (Mesulam et al., 1983) and also may modulate cortical activity (Buszaki et al., 1988). Bilateral excitotoxic lesions of the nucleus basalis magnocellularis enhanced spleen T cell mitogenesis and natural killer cell activity but did not modify B-cell mitogenesis and blood T-cell subset distribution (Cherkaoui et al., 1990). Left- or right-unilateral lesions however had no influence on these immunological parameters. The immunological effects of lesions of the nucleus basalis were studied shortly after lesioning, the increase in lymphocyte reactivity may be only transient and followed by depression. Further experiments performed at various time intervals are necessary to answer this question. The possible role of the various subcortical structures involved in the asymmetrical brain cortex of the immune system is a field wide open for further research.

The immunological effects of unilateral cortical lesions may be finally mediated by the autonomous nervous system and/or by hormones of the hypothalamo-pituitary axis. Previous studies have shown that plasma levels of ACTH and corticosterone were not modified 7 weeks after cortical lesions. These results are consistent with our data with mice, in which tissue lymphocyte distribution susceptible to corticoids was unchanged after hemicortical ablation (Barnéoud et al., 1990b). Prolactin levels in rats with unilateral ablation of right or left fronto-parieto-occipital cortex were similar to controls, although prolactin may be depressed after a lesion restricted to the parieto-occipital parts of the cortex (Lahoste et al., 1989). Following cortical ablations, however the hormonal response may precede alterations of immune reactivity. The latter may be observed when the hormone levels return to basal levels. A more complete study of the activity of both the hypothalamo-pituitary axis and the autonomous nervous system after cortical lesioning or depending on functional brain asymmetry is currently under investigations. Sex hormones do not appear to be involved in the immunological consequences of hemicortex ablations. Similar results have been observed for males and females (Barnéoud et al., 1987; Lahoste et al., 1989; Barnéoud et al., 1988b). By contrast, the association between paw-preference and immune reactivity is sex-dependent (Neveu et al., 1988; 1989; Betancur et al., 1990). As sex hormones are known to be involved in immune reactivity, auto-immune processes and brain development, they may also be important factors in the association between brain asymmetry and activity of the immune system.

As the central nervous system modulates immunity, it could be expected that the immune system communicates with the central nervous system. Indeed, animals immunized with sheep erythrocytes showed, at the peak of the plaque-forming cell response, enhanced electrical activity of neurons in the ventromedial hypothalamus (Besedovsky et al., 1977) and depressed turnover of norepinephrine in the hypothalamus and in the spleen (Besedovsky et al., 1983). On the other hand, recent findings suggest that interleukin-1 stimulates corticotropin releasing factor by the hypothalamus and, therefore increases levels of serum corticoids which have immunoregulatory functions. Thus, a complete loop between nervous and immune systems is likely evidenced. As the modulation of the immune system by the central nervous system may be lateralized the information sent by the immune system towards the central nervous system also should be processed asymmetrically. In fact, stimulation of the immune system by bacillus Calmette-Guérin, a good inducer of interleukin-1 production, increased norepinephrine levels in both hemispheres but significantly only in the right one. Furthermore, norepinephrine levels in the right hemisphere was correlated with the ability of lymphocytes to proliferate after mitogenic stimulation (Barnéoud et al., 1988c). Similarly, Freund's complete adjuvant induced an asymmetrical increase of ornithine decarboxylase activity in the brain (Neidhart and Larson, 1990).

In conclusion our studies suggest that the bidirectional connections between the central nervous system and the immune system may be lateralized. The mechanisms involved in the asymmetrical brain modulation of immune responses are currently under investigation.

Aknowledgement
I would like to thank Prof. G. Taylor for his critical review of the manuscript.

References

Barnéoud, P., Le Moal, M. & Neveu, P.J. (1990a). Asymmetrical distribution of brain monoamines in left- and right-handed mice. *Brain Research*, 1990, 520, 317-321.

Barnéoud, P., Le Moal, M. & Neveu, P.J. (1990b). Asymmetrical effects of cortical ablation on brain monoamines in mice. *Int. J. Neurosci.* in press.

Barnéoud, P., Neveu, P.J., Vitiello, S. & Le Moal M. (1987). Functional heterogeneity of the right and left cerebral neocortex in the modulation of the immune system. *Physiology and Behavior*, 41, 525-530.

Barnéoud, P., Neveu, P.J., Vitiello, S., & Le Moal, M. (1988a). Early effects of right or left cerebral cortex ablation on mitogen-induced spleen lymphocyte DNA-synthesis. *Neuroscience Letters*, 90, 302-307.

Barnéoud, P., Neveu, P.J., Vitiello, S. & Le Moal, M. (1990b). Lymphocyte homing after unilateral brain cortex ablation. *Immunology Letters*, 24, 223-227.

Barnéoud, P., Neveu, P.J., Vitiello, S., Mormède, P. & Le Moal, M. (1988b). Brain neocortex immunomodulation in rats. *Brain Research*, 474, 394-398.

Barnéoud, P., Rivet, J.M., Vitiello, S., Le Moal, M. & Neveu, P.J. (1988c). Brain norepinephrine levels after BCG stimulation of the immune system. *Immunology Letters*, 18, 201-204.

Bernton, E.W., Beach, J.F., Holaday, J.W., Smallbridge, R.C. & Fein, H.G. (1987). Release of multiple hormones by a direct action of interleukin-1 on pituitary cells. *Science*, 238, 519-521.

Besedovsky, H.O., Del Rey, A., Sorkin, E., Da Prada, M., Burri, R. & Honegger, C. (1983). The immune response evoques changes in brain noradrenergic neurons. *Science*, 221, 564-566.

Besedovsky, H.O., Sorkin, E., Felix, D. & Haas, H. (1977). Hypothalamic changes during the immune response. *European Journal of Immunology*, 7, 323-325.

Betancur, C., Neveu, P.J., Vitiello, S. & Le Moal, M. (1991). Natural killer cell activity is associated with brain asymmetry in male mice. *Brain Behav. Immun.*, in press.

Betancur, C., Velez, A., Cabanieu, R., Le Moal, M. & Neveu, P.J. (1990). Association between left-handedness and allergy: a reappraisal. *Neuropsychologia*, 28; 223-227.

Buszaki G., Bickford, R.G., Ponomareff, G., Thal, L.J., Mandel, R & Gage, F.H. (1988). Nucleus basalis and thalamic control of neocortical activity in the freely moving rat. *J. Neurosci.*, 8, 4007-4026.

Cherkaoui, J., Mayo, W., Neveu, P.J. Kelley, K.W., Dantzer, R., Le Moal, M. & Simon, H. (1990). The nucleus basalis is involved in brain modulation of the immune system in rats. *Brain Research,* 516, 345-348.

Collins, R.L. (1985). On the inheritance of direction and degree of asymmetry. In S.D. Glick (Ed.), *Cerebral lateralization in nonhuman species* (pp. 41-71). New York, Academic Press.

Cosi, V., Citterio, A. & Pasquino, C. (1988). A study of hand preference in myasthenia gravis. *Cortex*, 24, 573-577.

Cross, R.J. & Roszman, T.L. (1989). Neuroendocrine modulation of immune function, the role of prolactin. *Progress in Neuroendocrinoimmunology*, 2, 17-20.

Flor-Henry, P. (1976). Lateralized temporal-limbic dysfunction and psychopathology. *Annals NY Academy Sciences*, 280, 777-795.

Geschwind, N. & Behan, P. (1982). Left handedness: association with immune disease, migraine and developmental learning disorders. *Proceeding National Academy Science*, 79, 5097-5100.

Glick, S.D., Meibach, R.C., Cox, R.D. & Maayani, S. (1979). Multiple and interrelated functional asymmetries in rat brain. *Life Science*, 25, 395-400.

Glick, S.D., Ross, D. & Hough, L. (1982). Lateral asymmetry of neurotransmitters in human brain. *Brain Research*, 234, 53-63.

La Hoste, G.J., Neveu , P.J., Mormède, P., & Le Moal, M. (1989). Hemispheric asymmetries in the effects of cerebral cortical ablations on mitogen-induced lymphoproliferation and plasma prolactin levels in female rats. *Brain Research*, 483, 123-129.

Levy, J. (1974). Psychobiological implications of bilateral asymmetry. In: Hemisphere function in the human brain. Dimond, S.J. & Beaumont, J.G. (Eds.), *P. Elek*, London, 1974, pp. 121-183.

Maaser, B.W. & Farley, F.H. (1988). A review of left hemisphere dysfunction and hyperarousal and the effects of chlorpromazine in schizophrenics. *Research Communication Psycholology Psychiatry and Behavior*, 13, 177-192.

Mesulam, M.M.; Mufson, E.J., Wainer, B.H. & Levey A.I. (1983). Central cholinergic pathways in the rat: an overview based on an alternative nomenclature (Ch1-Ch6). *Neuroscience*, 10, 1185-1201.

Neidhart, M. & Larson, D.F. (1990). Freund's complete adjuvant induces ornithine decarboxylase activity in the central nervous system of male rats and triggers the release of pituitary hormones. *J. Neuroimmunol.*, 26, 97-105.

Neveu, P.J. (1988). Cerebral neocortex modulation of immune functions. *Life Science*, 42, 1917-1923.

Neveu, P.J., Barnéoud, P., Vitiello, S. & Le Moal, M. (1988a). Immune functions after bilateral neocortex ablation in mice. *Neuroscience Research Communication*, 3, 183-190.

Neveu, P.J., Barnéoud, P., Vitiello, S., Betancur C., & Le Moal, M. (1988b). Brain modulation of the immune system: association between lymphocyte responsiveness and paw preference in mice. *Brain Research*, 457, 392-394.

Neveu, P.J., Barnéoud, P., Georgiades, O., Vitiello, S., Vincendeau, P., & Le Moal, M. (1989a). Brain neocortex modulation of the mononuclear phagocytic system. *Journal of Neuroscience Research*, 22, 392-394.

Neveu, P.J., Betancur, C., Barnéoud, P., Preud'homme, J.L., Aucouturier, P., Le Moal, M. & Vitiello, S. (1989b). Functional brain asymmetry and murine systemic lupus erythematosus. *Brain Research*, 498, 159-162.

Neveu, P.J., Barnéoud, P., Vitiello, S., Kelley, K.W. & Le Moal, M. (1989c). Brain neocortex modulation of mitogen-induced interleukin-2, but not interleukin-1, production. *Immunology Letters*, 21, 307-310.

Neveu, P.J., Betancur, C., Barnéoud, P., Vitiello, S. & LeMoal, M. (1991). Functional brain asymmetry and lymphocyte proliferation in female mice: effects of left and right cortical ablation. Brain Res., 550, 125-128.

Neveu, P.J., Taghzouti, K., Dantzer, R., Simon, H. & Le Moal, M. (1986). Modulation of mitogen-induced lymphoproliferation by cerebral neocortex. *Life Science*, 38, 1907-1913.

Oke, A., Lewis, R. & Adams, R.N. (1980). Hemispheric asymmetry of norepinephrin distribution in rat thalamus. *Brain Research*, 188, 269-272.

Pennington, B.F., Smith, S.D., Kimberling, W.J., Green, P.A. & Haith, M.M. (1987). Left-handedness and immune disorders in familial dyslexics. *Archives of Neurology*, 44, 634-939.

Qiu-Shi, L. & Gui-Zhen, Y. (1987). Immunoregulatory effect of neocortex in mice. *Immunol. Invest.*, 16, 87-96.

Renoux, G. & Bizière, K. (1986). Brain neocortex lateralized control of immune recognition. *Integrative Psychiatry*, 4, 32-40.

Renoux, G. Bizière, K., Renoux, M., Guillaumin, J.M. & Degenne, D. (1983). A balanced brain asymmetry modulates T cell-mediated events. *J. Neuroimmunol.*, 5, 227-238.

Salcedo, J.R., Spiegler, B.J., Gibson, E. & Magilavy, D.B. (1985). The autoimmune disease systemic lupus erythematosus is not associated with left-handedness. *Cortex*, 21, 645-647.

Satz, P. & Soper, H.V. (1986). Left-handedness, dyslexia and autoimmune disorder: a critique. Journal Clinical Experimental Neuropsychology, 8, 453-458.

Wishaw, I.Q., O'Connor, W.T. & Dunnet, S.B. (1986). The contribution of motor cortex, nigrostriatal dopamine and caudate-putamen to skilled forelimb use in the rat. *Brain*, 109, 805-843.

Wofsy, D. (1984). Hormone, handedness and autoimmunity. *Immunology Today*, 5, 169-170.

Part II

Neuroendocrine Issues and Immunocompetence

Chapter 4

The Positive Regulation of T-Cells by the Neocortex is Likely to Involve a Dopamine Pathway

Gérard Renoux
Micheline Renuox

Immunological Laboratory
Faculty of Medicine
Tours, France

While studying the immunological consequences of injecting sodium diethyldithiocarbamate (dithiocarb, DTC, imuthiol ") into mice, we observed that the increase in T cell-mediated responses was delayed for a few days post treatment and that the anabolic influence on endotoxin-emaciated animals required a lag period of two weeks. This suggested to us the operation of a central form of control, possibly related to the CNS (Renoux & Renoux, 1979). Since both the hypothalamus and the autonomic nervous system receive inputs from various centres of the CNS, we therefore assumed that other regions of the CNS could be involved in the modulation of immunologic functions. A lateralized neocortical control of T-cell numbers and functions, not affecting B-cells, was indeed demonstrated (Renoux, Bizière, Renoux & Guillaumin, 1980a; Bizière, Guillaumin, Degenne, Bardos, Renoux & Renoux 1985; Renoux & Bizière, 1986). Recent findings also demonstrate that the immunostimulant activity of imuthiol is influenced by the neocortex (Renoux, Renoux, Bizière, Guillaumin, Bardos & Degenne, 1984; Renoux, 1988).

In addition, exploration of the possible pathways between the neocortex and the immune system has been conducted to show the role of dopamine [DA] (Renoux, Bizière, Renoux, Steinberg, Kan & Guillaumin, 1989).

At 6-8 weeks of age, C3H/HeJ female mice were randomly assigned to one of five surgical procedures under chloral hydrate anaesthesia: (a) right partial neocortical ablation; (b) left partial neocortical ablation; (c) partial bilateral neocortical ablation; (d) a sham operation, or (e) no surgery. Similar lesions, involving approximately one third of the fronto-parietal cortex without penetrating the corpus callosum, were performed on the left and right cerebral neocortex by shallow knife cuts (Bizière et al., 1985; Renoux et al., 1980a, 1983, 1984).

A 10-week interval between surgery and testing was observed to minimize the consequences of anaesthesia and surgical stress. Fifty to 100 mice from each of the randomly assigned groups were then tested in subgroups of 3-10 animals with assays that were reassessed over a period of more than 3 years to verify the repeatability of the findings. Samples were drawn between 9 and 9.30 a.m. to minimize circadian changes. Mice with a unilateral lesion as well as sham-operated and "no surgery" mice served as controls for symmetrically lesioned animals. No differences were ever observed between the two control groups of sham-operated and no surgery animals: the data were, therefore, pooled in a single control group.

Imuthiol was found to act specifically on the T-lymphocyte lineage through an increased synthesis of hepatosin by the liver. In addition, imuthiol exhibits a variety of pharmacologic activities as an antioxydant and free radical scavenger acting on the monooxygenase system; it is also a dopamine-ß-hydroxylase inhibitor (Renoux & Renoux, 1979; Renoux, 1982; Renoux, 1984; Renoux & Renoux,1984). The search for links between the cortex and the mediators of immunity induced us to evaluate the reciprocal influences of neocortex lesions and imuthiol on immune parameters.

The experimental procedures used were the same as those described above. Imuthiol was dissolved in pyrogen-free, sterile phosphate buffer, pH 7.2. A single dose (25 mg/kg-1) was administered subcutaneously in a volume of 0.2 ml, 10 weeks post surgery and 4 days prior to testing. Controls were treated with a s.c. injection of 0.2 ml buffer. Pyrogen-free syringes were used throughout. All administered suspensions were checked as being negative in the Limulus amoebocyte lysate gelation test to avoid the stimulant effect of endotoxin-like products.

Table 1 summarizes the findings. Collectively, these demonstrate that the drug is equally active in intact animals and in left-lesioned mice, is inactive in right-lesioned mice and only weakly active in bilaterally lesioned animals. A possible explanation for the findings could be that the left neocortex emits signals which antagonize the immunopotentiating effects of imuthiol and that in non-lesioned animals the right neocortex inhibits the left neocortex.

Tab. 1: Effects of partial neocortical lesions on immune parameters and imuthiol-induced stimulation.

Immune parameters	Right Saline	Right Imuthiol	Left Saline	Left Imuthiol	None Imuthiol
	Lesions and Treatment				
Spleen T-cell number	+	=	-	+	+
MHC antigens on T-cells	+	=	-	+	+
T-cell responses to mitogens and antigens	+	=	-	+	+
T-cell response to alloantigens	+	+	-	+	+
T-cell-specific serum activity	+	=	-	+	+
Natural Killer cell activity	0	+	-	+	+
Spleen B-cell number	0	0	0	0	0
B-cell responses to mitogens and antigens	0	0	0	0	0
Macrophage cytotoxic response	0	0	0	0	0

+ Increase or - decrease in comparison to unlesioned and untreated controls; = a response similar to that of lesioned and saline treated controls; 0 a response similar to that of unlesioned controls. Results from bilateral lesions are not shown, as they resemble those of left-lesioned animals (Renoux et al. 1987).

Thus, treatment with imuthiol confirms that a major hemispheric asymmetry modulates T-cell maturational processes and T-cell-mediated events, suggesting a strong inhibition of the left neocortex by the right neocortex, particularly with regard to the specific action of imuthiol on the T-cell lineage.

Present results not only show the cerebral neocortex to be involved in T-cell recruitment and activation but also that the phenomenon is lateralized. Hemispheric lateralization is present at a population level in female C3H/HeJ mice. If it were present at the individual level, the effect would be randomly distributed. Furthermore and, importantly, our findings extend to a neocortical level the observation that the involvement of the CNS in drug response may be asymmetrical. MPTP (1-methyl-4-phenyl-1,2,3,6-tetrahydropyridine) is a neurotoxicant that provokes severe degeneration of the dopaminergic nigrostriatal pathway. Since dopamine metabolism, immune regulation, and cerebral laterality seem to be disturbed in diseases such as schizophrenia or Parkinson's disease, we thought it of interest to determine whether MPTP affects mouse immune responses and whether imuthiol can modify the MPTP-induced changes (Renoux, Bizière, Renoux, Steinberg, Kan & Guillaumin, 1989).

As shown in Tables 2 to 4, MPTP modifies the immune system in Swiss Webster mice by reducing T-lymphocyte percentage and function and increasing B-cell number and activity. A moderate dose (25 mg/kg) of imuthiol selectively increases T-cell-dependent responses, confirming previous findings with other mouse strains. It also enhances striatal DA and metabolite levels in control animals. Imuthiol restores T-lymphocyte levels and activities, but only the DA level, in MPTP-treated mice. Since imuthiol passes the blood-brain barrier (Guillaumin, Lepape & Renoux, 1986), the restoration of immune activities and partial protection against MPTP neurotoxicity might be due to an in situ effect of imuthiol. Imuthiol reduces the brain level of the toxic metabolite, methyl-4-phenylpyridinium ion [MPP^+], through its protective influence against chemicals (Renoux, 1982).

Tab. 2: Influences of imuthiol on the MPTP-induced fall in striatal dopamine and metabolite levels.

Treatment	% of control levels[a]			
	DA	DOPAC	HVA	3-MT
MPTP	56 ± 4*	25 ± 3*	47 ± 7*	50 ± 4*
Imuthiol	134 ± 17	138 ± 14	133 ± 9	146 ± 12*
MPTP + imuthiol	86 ± 8	34 ± 5*	56 ± 4*	65 ± 5*

Striatal amine levels (µg/g) in controls (5 mice); dopamine (DA), 5.94 ± 0.209; 3,4-dihydroxyphenyl acetic acid (DOPAC), 0.806 ± 0.074; homovanillic acid (HVA), 0.520 ± 0.053; 3-metoxytyramine (3-MT), 0.387 ± 0.028.

[a] Means ± SEM for 5 mice individually tested in each experimental group.
* p < 0.01 to controls.

Tab. 3: Influences of MPTP and imuthiol on spleen lymphocyte populations.

Treatment	Tests		
	Total spleen cells (x 10^6)	Thy-1+%	B(sig+) %
Controls	134 ± 46	22.1 ± 2.4	49.4 ± 2.6
MPTP	165 ± 33	17.0 ± 1.2*	56.6 ± 3.5*
Imuthiol	125 ± 37	25.2 ± 0.8*	42.6 ± 2.0*
MPTP + imuthiol	162 ± 39	22.3 ± 0.5	44.8 ± 7.4

Mean values of three experiments, each involving 5 mice, individually tested in triplicate assays. * significantly different from control values ($p \leq 0.01$).

Tab. 4.: Influences of MPTP and imuthiol on lymphoproliferative responses.

Test	Treatment			
	Controls	MPTP	Imuthiol	MPTP + Imuthiol
No mitogen	1.5 ± 0.5	3.0 ± 0.8	1.1 ± 0.6	5.1 ± 0.8*
PHA[a]	56 ± 6	53 ± 6	72 ± 7*	117 ± 5*
ConA[a]	106 ± 4	85 ± 9*	147 ± 7*	124 ± 6*
PWM[a]	33 ± 7	48 ± 6*	34 ± 4	29 ± 1
MLC[b]	13 ± 0.5	4.2 ± 0.1*	18 ± 0.2*	12.3 ± 0.4

[a] Net cpm (induced - spontaneous) ± S.E.M. of [^{3}H]thymidine incorporation of triplicate cultures from four mice, individually tested in each experimental group.
[b] % labeled thymidine uptake by equal numbers of spleen cells from control and treated Swiss Webster mice stimulated with a pool of irradiated lymphocytes from six different mouse strains.

* significantly different from control values ($p \leq 0.05$).

The data obtained in MPTF- and imuthiol-treated mice indirectly confirm that brain structures control the T-lymphocyte arm of the immune system and suggest that dopamine may play an important role. They provide additional support for the suggestion that the catecholamines have a regulatory effect on the activities of the immune system. A specific DA receptor is described in thymocytes and splenocytes (Ovadia & Abramsky, 1987). A brain neocortex asymmetry controls T-cell recruitment and activity, and the imuthiol-induced stimulation. Lateral asymmetries are known in striatal DA receptors (Schneider, Murphy & Coons, 1982) and for DA concentration in the cortex (Rosen, Finklestein, Stoll, Yutzey & Denenberg, 1984). Altogether, the findings strongly suggest that DA could be among the neurotransmitters involved in pathways from the neocortex for T-cell recruitment and activities, as was recently confirmed by Devoino et al. (1988). Our results demonstrate unequivocally that the neocortex influences T-cell-mediated events and controls the mechanisms of action of imuthiol. T-cell recruitment, number and function, including NK activity, as well as the production of a specific serum factor in normal animals, depend on a balanced brain asymmetry in which the right hemisphere controls the inductive influence of signals emitted by the left hemisphere. Partial brain lesions do not directly affect B-cells or macrophages. Furthermore, treatment with imuthiol reveals discrete, differential influences of the neocortex on T-cell activities. The immunopotentiating effects of imuthiol do not require an intact neocortex, but appear to be subject to a negative control from the left hemisphere, which is in turn inhibited by the right hemisphere.

The immune and central nervous systems display striking similarities. Both systems show a remarkable degree of cell diversity; both possess memory characteristics which do not exist in other systems. Both cellular systems share in common antigens which are lacking in all the other cells tested. Both systems serve functions of adaptation, defense, and homeostasis, and both relate the organism to an often hostile environment.

Cell-to-cell learning in both systems and communication between brain and body involve an intricate network in which messages are transmitted and received. The present findings strongly suggest an important role of dopamine in transmitting these signals.

Lateralization for immune recognition and cognitive processes is an attribute of cortical brain structures. Both systems are interconnected to allow quick adaptation for those unpredictable changes that are far too rapid for evolutionary adaptation to take place.

Our results, based on a large array of immunologic testing, clearly show that the neocortex controls the immune system, whatever the pathways involved might be. They demonstrate also that a lateralized neocortical function can be involved in the activities of pharmacological agents. That imuthiol, a sulphur-containing agent of low molecular weight, requires the mediation of the neocortex to increase T-cell number and function could provide a potent link for renewed investigations of the pathways by which the CNS participates in regulation of the immune system. Further studies will hopefully enhance our understanding of the mechanisms mediating these reciprocal effects. This may well afford the opportunity to develop new compounds acting on the immune system. Progress in these research areas may well supply yet unexpected advances in etiologies, therapies, and even in the diagnosis of immune-based diseases and cancer, and neuroendocrine or psychopathologic disorders.

References

Bizière, K., Guillaumin, J.M., Degenne, D., Bardos, P., Renoux, M. & Renoux, G. (1985). Lateralized neocortical modulation of the T-cell lineage. In: Guillemin, R., Cohn, M., Melnechuk, T. (Eds.) *Neural modulation of immunity*. Raven Press, New York, pp. 81-94.

Devoino, L., Alperina, E. & Idova, G. (1988). Dopaminergic stimulation of the immune reaction: interaction of serotoninergic and dopaminergic systems in neuroimmunomodulation. *International Journal of Neuroscience* 40:271-288.

Guillaumin, J.M., Lepape, A. & Renoux, G. (1986). Fate and distribution of radioactive sodium diethyldithiocarbamate (Imuthiol ") in the mouse. *International Journal of Immunopharmacology* 8:859-865.

Ovadia, H. & Abramsky, O. (1987). Dopamine receptors on isolated membranes of rat lymphocytes. *Journal of Neuroscience Research* 18:70-74.

Renoux, G. (1982). Immunopharmacologie et pharmacologie du diethyldithiocarbamate (DTC). *Journal de Pharmacologie* (Paris) 13 Suppl. 1:95-134.

Renoux, G. (1983). The thymic factor system. *Biomedicine and Pharmacotherapy* 37:433-440.

Renoux, G. (1984). The mode of action of imuthiol (sodium diethyldithiocarbamate). A new role for the brain neocortex and the endocrine liver in the regulation of the T-cell lineage. In: Fenichel, R.L. & Chirigos, M.A. (Eds.) *Immune modulation agents and their mechanisms of action*. Marcel Dekker, New York, pp. 607-624.

Renoux, G. (1988). The cortex regulates the immune system and the activities of a T-cell specific immunopotentiator. *International Journal of Neuroscience* 39:177-187.

Renoux, G. & Bizière, K. (1986). Brain neocortex lateralized control of immune recognition. *Integrative Psychiatry* 4:32-40.

Renoux, G. & Bizière, K. (1987). Asymmetrical involvement of the cerebral neocortex in the response to an immunopotentiator, sodium diethyldithiocarbamate. *Journal of Neuroscience Research* 18:230-238.

Renoux, G., Bizière, K., Bardos, P., Degenne, D. & Renoux, M. (1982). NK activity in mice is controlled by the brain neocortex. In: Herberman ,R.B. (Ed.) *NK cells and other natural effector cells.*. Academic Press, New York, pp. 639-643.

Renoux, G., Bizière, K., Renoux, M. & Guillaumin, J.M. (1980). Le cortex cerebral régle les réponses immunes des souris. *Comptes Rendus de l'Académie des Sciences (Paris)* 290D:719-722.

Renoux, G., Bizière, K., Renoux, M. & Guillaumin, J.M. (1982). Neocortical lateralization of the production of T cell-inducing factors in mice. *Scandinavian Journal of Immunology* 17:45-50.

Renoux, G., Bizière, K., Renoux, M., Guillaumin, J.M. & Degenne, D. (1983). A balanced brain asymmetry modulates T-cell-mediated events. *Journal of Neuroimmunology* 5:227-238.

Renoux, G., Bizière, K., Renoux, M., Bardos, P. & Degenne, D. (1987). Consequences of bilateral brain neocortex ablation in imuthiol-induced immunostimulation in mice. In: Jankovic, B.D., Spector, N.H. & Markovic, B.M. (Eds.). *Neuroimmune interactions.*. Academy of Sciences, New York, Vol. 496, pp. 346-353.

Renoux, G., Bizière, K., Renoux, M., Steinberg, R., Kan, J.P. & Guillaumin, J.M. (1989). Sodium diethyldithiocarbamate protects against the MPTP-induced inhibition of immune responses in mice. *Life Science* 44:771-777.

Renoux, G. & Renoux, M. (1979). Immunopotentiation and anabolism induced by sodium diethyldithiocarbamate. *Journal of Immunopharmacology* 1:247-267.

Renoux, G. & Renoux, M. (1982). Hepatosin. *International Journal of Immunopharmacology* 4:300.

Renoux, G. & Renoux, M. (1984). Diethyldithiocarbamate (DTC). A biological augmenting agent specific for T-cells. In: Fenichel, R.L. & Chirigos, M.A. (Eds.) *Immune modulation agents and their mechanisms*. Marcel Dekker, New York, pp. 7-20.

Renoux, G., Renoux, M. & Bizière, K. (1988). Brain neocortex and imuthiol regulate the expression of MHC antigens in mouse T-lymphocytes. *Immunopharmacology and Immunotoxicology* 10:219-229.

Renoux, G., Renoux, M., Bizière, K., Guillaumin, J.M., Bardos, P. & Degenne, D. (1984). Involvement of brain neocortex and liver in the regulation of T-cells: The mode of action of sodium diethlydithiocarbamate (DTC). *Immunopharmacology* 7:89-100.

Rosen, G.D., Finklstein, S., Stoli, A.L., Yutzey, D.A. & Denenberg, V.H. (1984). Neurochemical asymmetries in the albino rat's cortex, striatum, and nucleus accumbens. *Life Sciences* 34:1143-1148.

Schneider, L.H., Murphy, R.B. & Coons, E.E. (1982). Lateralization of striatal dopamine (D2) receptors in normal rats. *Neuroscience Letters* 33:281-284.

Chapter 5

Corticosteroids as Modulators of Sensory Processing in Man

Gabriele Fehm-Wolfsdorf*
Jan Born
Dethart Nagel
Helmuth Zenz
Horst Lorenz Fehm

Department of Medical Psychology
Department of Internal Medicine I
University of Ulm, F.R.G.
*present address: Psychological Institut,
University of Kiel, F.R.G.

Introduction

Glucocorticoids play an important role in interactions between the endocrine, immune, and central nervous systems, enabling integrative higher functions for behavioural adaptation. Humoral efferences have been extensively studied to elucidate the role glucocorticoids play in stressful situations. The hypothalamic-pituitary-adrenal (HPA) axis is involved in complex functioning aimed to maintain homeostasis in the face of a constantly changing internal and external environment. According to Tausk (1970) and Munck et al. (1984) glucocorticoids prevent the primary defense responses to stress from overshooting. Defense mechanisms, for example, the release of epinephrine, prostaglandines, lymphokines, might become damaging for the organism if they were not controlled by glucocorticoid actions. If coping with stress fails, an elevated level of circulating glucocorticoids persists. Particularly in limbic structures, persistently high glucocorticoid levels in conditions of chronic stress are thought to induce neuronal degeneration and cell loss resembling the degenerative changes during aging (Sapolski et al., 1986).

Little attention has been given to the physiology of the afferent glucocorticoid system. As well as any other cells of the organism, brain cells represent a target for hormonal actions. Glucocorticoids easily pass through the blood-brain-barrier and express their information by binding to specific receptors within the brain. The brain seems to be the only tissue with two different glucocorticoid receptors (McEwen et al., 1986; DeKloett & Reul, 1987). A mineralocorticoid (Type I) and a glucocorticoid (Type II) receptor have been identified.

The Type I receptor probably mediates mineralocorticoid action in circumventricular organs, but has a role as physiological glucocorticoid receptor in limbic structures, mainly in the hippocampus. The limbic Type I receptor responds with stringent specificity to corticosterone or cortisol, depending on the species. Via this receptor system glucocorticoids are assumed to control basal activity of the HPA-axis, to affect the magnitude of the response to sensory input and to coordinate circadian events like sleep and food intake (for a review: DeKloett & Reul, 1987). Compared to Type I, the Type II receptor has a 10-fold lower affinity to natural glucocorticoid, whereas synthetic glucocorticoids such as dexamethasone bind with very high affinity to Type II receptors. Type II receptors are found to be widely distributed throughout the brain, both in neurons and glial cells. Via Type II receptors glucocorticoids exert a negative feedback action on stress-induced HPA-activity, restore homeostasis and control adaptation (DeKloett & Reul, 1987). This holds for rat brain; differential CNS-receptor systems in man, however, have rarely been studied till now.

Differential effects of hydrocortisone and dexamethasone on sleep have been described recently in man (Fehm et al., 1986; Born et al., 1987). The present series of experiments aimed to differentiate the effects of hydrocortisone and dexamethasone on sensory processing. In patients with adrenal cortical insufficiency, lacking endogenous cortisol secretion, Henkin and co-workers (Henkin et al., 1963; Henkin et al., 1967; Henkin, 1975) observed a marked increase in the patients' sensitivity to taste, olfactory, and auditory stimuli. Glucocorticoid substitution therapy was able to normalize these aberrations. In healthy subjects Henkin (1975) observed considerable circadian changes in detection acuity, paralleling the circadian rhythm of cortisol secretion, with maximum values in the morning and lowest secretion during the evening hours. He concluded that there were physiological oscillations in cortisol modulate sensory functions. Consequently, cortisol release in stressful situations is expected to reduce the amount of incoming information and may thus help the organism to cope more efficiently with the stressor.

The present studies tested taste detection acuity, adopting Henkin's methodology (Henkin et al., 1963), and various other auditory functions. Experiments were performed in the morning as well as in the evening to elucidate at the same time circadian influences. Pretreatment of patients in the experimental sessions included administration of hydrocortisone, which is equivalent to the endogenous cortisol and has glucocorticoid and mineralocorticoid properties, dexamethasone, a synthetic pure glucocorticoid, and spironolactone, a mineralocorticoid-antagonist, to differentiate effects mediated via different steroid receptor systems.

Material and methods

We here summarize four experiments (A, B, C, D), two of which have been described in more detail elsewhere (Fehm-Wolfsdorf et al., 1989; Fehm-Wolfsdorf et al., 1991). Table 1 gives an overview of subjects, tasks, and treatments in these studies.

Tab. 1 : Design and procedure of all studies (for details see text).

Study	No of Subjects	No of Sessions, Time of Day	Treatments	Tasks
A	15	3 morning	hydrocortisone, dexamethasone, placebo	taste detection acuity, mood
B	18	4 morning or evening	hydrocortisone, placebo	taste detection acuity, memory
C	15	3 morning	hydrocortisone, dexamethasone, placebo	auditory perception
D	13	4 evening	hydrocortisone, dexamethasone, spironolactone, placebo	auditory perception

In all studies, subjects were male student volunteers, non-smokers, who had given their written consent to participate in three or four experimental sessions, respectively, which were spaced one week apart.

Sessions of study A and C were scheduled at 9.00 h, study D included sessions at 18.00 h only. In study B half of the sessions took place in the morning, the other half in the evening. All studies were designed according to within-subject crossover double-blind designs to assess the effects of different treatments or time of day, respectively. Oral treatments consisted of 50 mg hydrocortisone, 2 mg dexamethasone, 200 mg spironolactone, and the respective placebo medications. With regard to the different half-lives and pharmacokinetics of these substances, intake of hydrocortisone was scheduled one hour prior to testing, whereas dexamethasone or spironolactone was administered nine hours prior.

Taste detection acuity was determined using a forced-choice task described by Henkin et al. (1963). A drop of NaCl solution and two drops of distilled water were put on the foremost third of the subject's tongue in random order. The subject was to decide immediately which of the three drops tasted salty and to rate on a five-point Likert scale how sure he was of his decision. Each of seven different concentrations were applied six times in random order (Fig. 1). The concentrations chosen were identical to those used by Henkin. Taste detection acuity was determined by the relative frequency (i.e. probability) of correct responses for a particular concentration of NaCl.

Mood was assessed by a check list of common German adjectives, the Eigenschaftswörterliste (EWL; Janke & Debus, 1978). For every item subjects had to decide whether the adjective described his present state of mood or not. Items were comprised of six dimensions. Changes in mood states have been reported in patients chronically treated with glucocorticoids (von Zerssen, 1976).

Memory performance consisted of a free recall task with immediate written recall. Materials included lists of 15 common German monosyllabic nouns which were presented as a tape-recording. In each session five different lists were used. Memory performance was scored as the probability of recall of the items on a list. This memory recall task was included in the investigation as an indicator of higher cognitive functioning which might be secondarily influenced if detection of incoming information were modulated by hormonal treatments.

Auditory perception tests should assess processing of stimuli at different levels of complexity. They included measurement of stapedial reflex to pure sinusoidal tones and noise at ipsi- and contralateral ears, pure tone audiogram at frequencies from 500 to 8000 hz, speech audiogram including responses to words and numbers, and brain stem evoked response audiometry (BERA). BERA was recorded using rarefaction clicks of 90 dB, 60 dB, and 40 dB/HL presented at a rate of 30 clicks/sec.

Cortisol was determined from blood and/or saliva samples to control for the effects of medication on endogenous cortisol secretion. Samples were drawn at the beginning, middle, and end of a session in most of the studies. Statistical analysis based on analyses of variance (ANOVA, BMDP2V) including repeated measures of TREATMENT and TIME OF DAY factors were performed.

Tab. 2:. Summary of Results.

Study	Dependent Variable	T	H	T x S
A	taste detection acuity	**	--	--
	detection of differences in taste	*	--	--
	mood scale	ns	--	--
B	taste detection acuity	ns	ns	--
	memory recall	ns	+	--
C	stapedial reflex	*	--	**
	pure tone audiogram	ns	--	ns
	speech audiogram	ns	--	--
	brain stem evoked responses	ns	--	--
D	stapedial reflex	+	--	*
	pure tone audiogram	ns	--	--
	speech audiogram	ns	--	--
	brain stem evoked responses	ns	--	--

T = ANOVA main effect of TREATMENT
H = ANOVA main effect for TIME OF DAY
T x S = ANOVA interaction between TREATMENT and STIMULUS QUALITY
+ = $p < 0.10$
* = $p < 0.05$
** = $p < 0.01$
ns = not significant
-- = not evaluated

Results

Table 2 summarizes the main results from all experiments. In detail, the following changes were observed:

Cortisol: Plasma and saliva cortisol levels confirmed the effectiveness of the treatment conditions and for placebo conditions showed the usual circadian differences. Plasma and saliva cortisol levels were highly correlated (in experiment B: r = 0.82). Fig. 1 shows mean cortisol levels in Experiment B as an example. Cortisol levels after intake of dexamethasone were very low; in Experiment A, for example, the mean plasma concentration was 0.5 µg/dl and the mean saliva

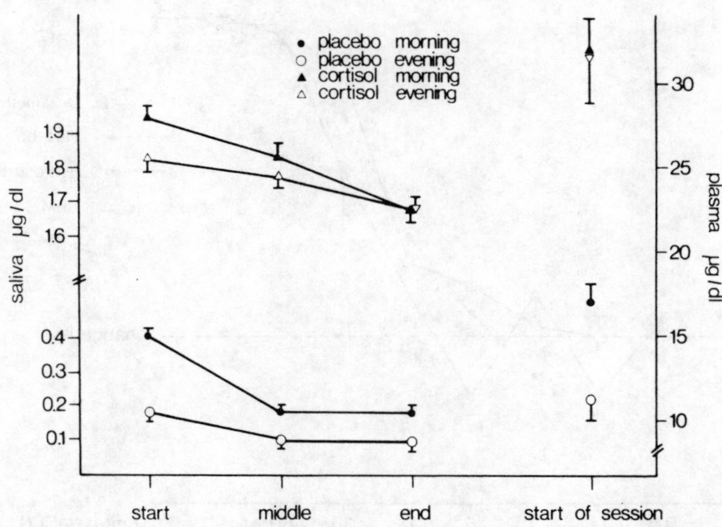

Fig. 1: Cortisol levels (mean and SEM) in plasma and saliva are given following intake of 50 mg hydrocortisone one hour prior to the experiment or placebo in the morning at 9.00 h or in the evening at 18.00 h (from 12.)

concentration 0.08 μg/dl. These effects appeared as statistically significant main effects for TREATMENT or TIME OF DAY. Cortisol levels decreased significantly from start to end of the sessions. This underlines that task performance per se was not stressful for our subjects.

Taste detection: The probability of correct responses in the forced-choice detection task varied between chance level at salt concentrations below 6 mM/L and always correct responses at the highest salt concentrations. Fig. 1 shows the effects of different treatments in Experiment A on taste detection acuity. Intake of hydrocortisone as compared to dexamethasone or placebo significantly reduced the probability of correct responses to stimuli in the threshold range between 6 mM/L and 30 mM/L NaCl. This effect, however, could not be replicated in Experiment B, including sessions in the morning and in the evening. Hydrocortisone in this study had no effect on detection performance compared to a placebo condition; however, a

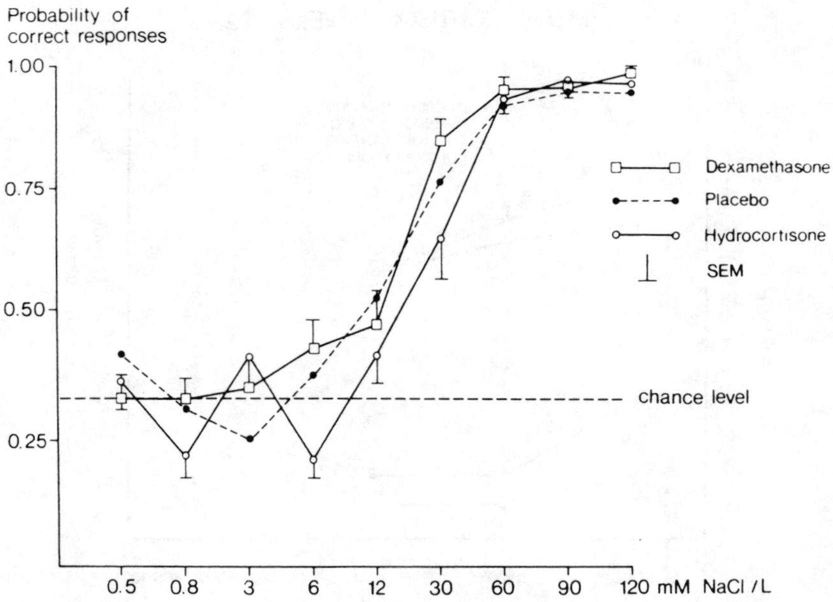

Fig. 2: Probability of correct responses across trials with different concentrations of NaCl following different treatments. After intake of hydrocortisone, correct responses in threshold range (6 to 30 mM/L) were significantly reduced compared to dexamethasone. Means and SEM are given (from 11).

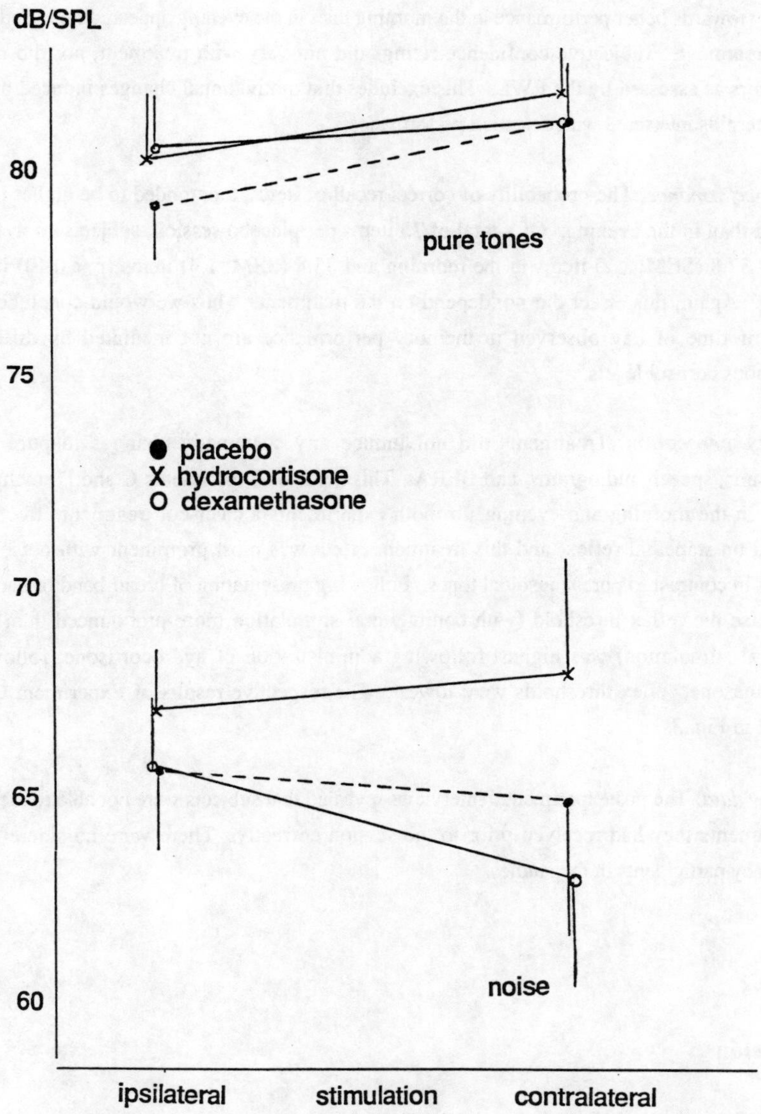

Fig. 3: Mean intensities (+SEM) sufficient to elicit the stapedial reflex of pure tones or noise for the different treatment conditions. Hydrocortisone significantly increases reflex threshold, particularly with contralateral ears.

tendency towards better performance in the morning than in the evening appeared independently of the treatment. Subjective confidence ratings did not vary with treatment, nor did mood parameters as assessed by the EWL. This excludes that motivational changes induced by the corticosteroids interfered with detection performance.

Recall performance: The probability of correct recall of items, too, tended to be higher in the morning than in the evening. Of a total of 75 items per placebo session, subjects on average recalled 37.8 (SEM: 1.2) items in the morning and 35.8 (SEM: 1.4) items ($p < 0.10$) in the evening. Again, this effect did not depend on the treatment. Thus we would conclude that effects of time of day observed in memory performance are not mediated by different endogenous cortisol levels.

Auditory perception: Treatments did not induce any systematic changes in pure tone audiograms, speech audiograms, and BERA. This held for Experiments C and D, including testings in the morning and evening. In both experiments a clear-cut treatment effect was obtained on stapedial reflex, and this treatment effect was most prominent with noise as a stimulus in contrast to pure sinusoidal tones. Following presentation of broad-band or narrow-band noise the reflex threshold (with contralateral stimulation more pronounced than with ipsilateral stimulation) was highest following administration of hydrocortisone; following dexamethasone, reflex thresholds were lowest. The respective results of Experiment C are depicted in Fig. 3.

Interview data: The postexperimental interviews revealed that subjects were not able to identify the treatments they had received prior to the session correctly. There were no side-effects reported by participants in the studies.

Discussion

Four studies in healthy volunteers aimed to elucidate afferent influences of glucocorticoids on sensory processing. We studied the influences of different hormones as well as the impact of the time of day associated with different endogenous cortisol levels. The pattern of results from all studies does not speak for glucocorticoid effects in normal man that are comparable to those observed by Henkin (1975) in patients with adrenocortical insufficiency. Nearly all variables varied with time of day, but the performance decreases in the evening cannot be attributed to glucocorticoid actions, as these effects did not depend on treatment conditions. However, pharmacologically induced changes of cortisol levels, being much clearer than circadian changes, modulated sensory processing in the same way as in patients with adrenocortical insufficiency: with high cortisol levels, subjects made more errors in taste detection and more intense stimulation was needed to evoke reflexes.

Some of our results are in contrast to Henkin's (1975) findings and hypotheses. However, his hypotheses on the physiological role of glucocorticoids were mainly based on studies in patients suffering from chronic hypo- or hypercortisolism. In chronic states regulation of glucocorticoid receptors may be changed, and more dramatic modulations of sensory functions may develop. Studies by Henkin's group in healthy volunteers on the same matter lack simultaneous determination of actual cortisol concentration and sensory acuity and hence may not provide a sufficient data base concerning normal physiology.

The most prominent effect in our studies was the modulation of the stapedial reflex to noise by different corticosteroids. Differential effects of hydrocortisone and dexamethasone may be hints to the involvement of Type I glucocorticoid receptors in the regulation of this reflex. Stumpf and Sar (1973) provided evidence for a wide distribution of steroid hormone receptors in the midbrain and spinal cord and suggested an important role of steroid hormones in the extrahypothalamic neuroendocrine, sensory and motor systems. In rat brain, Type I receptors are most densely present in brain stem motor nuclei (de Kloet, personal communication). Since the presence of receptors is essential for a hormone to act, the differential modulation of the stapedial reflex by steroids may hint at the existence of dual receptors in human midbrain areas. Since differential effects of dexamethasone and endogenous glucocorticoids have also been reported on serotonin release, the changes in stapedial reflex may involve serotonergic transmission.

To summarize, our results speak for the differential effects of glucocorticoids on sensory functioning in man. In the light of these findings, it appears to be interesting to study sensory changes under conditions of chronic stress with dramatically increased cortisol levels: if sensory functions during stress are distorted, a positive feedback loop between cortisol secretion and cognitive coping with the situation could develop hindering appropriate adaptation. Thus, the quality of cognitive coping processes in a stressful situation may be seen as an intervening variable in research on neuroendocrine-immune reactions to various stressors.

References

Born, J., Zwick, A., Roth, G., Fehm-Wolfsdorf, G. & Fehm, H.L. (1987). Differential effects of hydrocortisone, fluocortolone, and aldosterone on nocturnal sleep in humans. *Acta Endocrinol.*116:129.

De Kloet, E.R. & Reul, J.M.H.M. (1987). Feedback action and tonic influence of Corticosteroids on brain function: a concept arising from the heterogeneity of brain receptor systems. *Psychoneuroendocrinology* 12:83.

Fehm, H.L., Benkowitsch, R., Kern, W., Fehm-Wolfsdorf, G., Pauschinger P. & Born, J. (1986). Influences of corticosteroids, dexamethasone and hydrocortisone on sleep in humans. *Neuropsychobiology* 16:198.

Fehm-Wolfsdorf, G., Reutter, K., Zenz, H., Born, J. & Fehm, H.L. Stress hormones as modulators of perception (submitted).

Fehm-Wolfsdorf, G., Scheible, E., Zenz, H., Born ,J. & Fehm ,H.L. (1989).Taste thresholds in man are differentiallly influenced by hydrocortisone and dexamethasone. *Psychoneuroendocrinology*, 14:433.

Henkin, R.I. (1975). The role of adrenal corticosteroids in sensory processes. In: Greep, R.O. & Astwood, E.B. (Eds.). *Handbook of Physiology*. American Physiological Society, Washington.

Henkin, R.I., Gill, J.R. & Bartter, F.C. (1963). Studies on taste thresholds in normal man and in patients with adrenal cortical insufficiency: The role of sdrenal cortical steroids and of serum sodium concentration. *J. Clin. Invest.* 42:727.

Henkin, R.I., McGlone, R.E., Daly, R. & Bartter, F.C. (1967). Studies in auditory thresholds in normal man and in patients with adrenal cortical insufficiency: The role of adrenal cortical steroids. *J. Clin. Invest.* 46:429.

Janke W. & Debus G. (1978). Die Eigenschaftswörterliste. Hogrefe, Göttingen.

McEwen, B.S., De Kloet, E.R. & Rostene, W.H. (1986). Adrenal steroid receptors and actions in the nervous system. *Physiol. Rev.* 66:1121.

Munck, A., Guyre, P.M. & Holbrook, N.J. (1984). Physiological functions of glucocorticoids in stress and their relation to pharmacological actions. *Endocrine Rev*. 5:25.

Sapolski, R.M., Krey, L.C. & McEwen, B.S. (1986). The neuroendocrinology of stress and aging: The glucocorticoid cascade hypothesis. *Endocrine Rev*. 7:284.

Stumpf, W.E. & Sar, M. (1973). Steroid hormone target cells in the extrahypothalamic brain stem and spinal cord: Neuroendocrine significance. *J. Steroid. Biochem*. 11:801.

Tausk, M. (1970). *Pharmakologie der Hormone*. Thieme Verlag, Stuttgart.

Von Zerssen, D. (1976). Mood and behavioral changes under corticosteroid therapy. In: Itil, T.M., Laudahn, G. & Herrmann, W.M. (Eds.). *Psychotropic Actions of Hormones*. Spectrum Publications, New York.

Chapter 6

Effect of Repeated Stress and the Treatment with Ergot-Alkaloid Dihydroergosine on the Immune Response of Rats

Milivoj Boranic
Danka Pericic
Lidija Smejkal-Jagar
Nela Pivac

Department of Experimental Biology and Medicine
Rudjer Boskovic Institute
Zagreb, Yougoslavia

Introduction

Stressful conditions interfere with the immune response (reviewed, e.g. in Balitzky et al., 1983; Boranic et al., 1989; Dantzer & Kelley, 1989; Fox & Newberry 1984; Laudenslager 1983; Monjan, 1981; Shavit et al., 1985; Sklar & Anisman, 1981; Solomon et al,.1974). This has been attributed to an activation of the hypothalamo-pituitary-suprarenal axis (Gisler, 1973; Solomon et al., 1974) via central adrenergic, serotoninergic and, possibly, GABAergic mechanisms (Boranic et al., 1989; Culman et al., 1980; Dantzer & Kelley, 1989; Devino et al., 1986; Glavin, 1985; Kuriyama et al., 1983; Lenox et al., 1980; Okimura et al., 1986; Tuomisto & Männistö, 1986), resulting in hormonal changes that probably alter the organ distribution, proportions and reactivity of lymphocyte populations (Devoino et al., 1986; Okimura & Nigo, 1986; Okimura et al., 1986). Mechanisms bypassing the axis, such as neural transmission, opioid and other peptides, have been recognized more recently (Besedovsky et al., 1986; Blalock & Smith, 1985; Dantzer & Kelley, 1989; Kadlecova et al., 1987; Keller et al., 1983; Laudenslager, 1983; Shavit et al., 1985; Walker & Codd, 1985; Wibran, 1985), together with a feedback influence of the immune system on neuroendocrine regulation (Besedovsky et al., 1986; Blalock & Smith, 1985; Dantzer & Kelley, 1989;). Drugs affecting central and/or peripheral transmission of nerve signals may modulate the immune response in a way that either resembles or counteracts the effects of stress (Boranic et al., 1989; Cheido et al., 1987; Dadhich et al., 1980; Dantzer & Kelley, 1989; Devino et al., 1986; Gisler et al., 1971; Jackson et al., 1985; Martindupan & Dayer, 1982; Pierpaoli & Maestroni, 1978 a,b; Raskova et al., 1987; Rehulka, 1988) .

This preliminary communication describes the effects of dihydroergosine, a naturally occurring ergot-alkaloid (DHESN), on the immune response of animals subjected to repeated stress. This substance is a derivative of (+)lysergic acid with (3)5R,8R-configuration, having a pronounced hypotensive effect, attributable to its antagonism of noradrenaline at the postsynaptic level (Radulovic et al., 1984; Susic et al., 1984), and central serotoninergic effects affecting behaviour in a manner resembling imipramine (Manev & Pericic, 1988; Manev et al., 1989; Pericic & Manev, 1988), a classical antidepressant. It is an antagonist of serotoninergic-2 receptors (5-HT2R) (Mück-Seler & Pericic, 1989; Pericic, 1989; Pericic & Manev 1988; Pericic & Mück-Seler, 1990). GABAergic transmission is also affected by DHESN (Manev et al., 1989; Pericic & Manev, 1989).

Materials and Methods

Animals. Female Wistar rats from our colony, 8 to 10 weeks old and weighing 160 to 250 g, were used. They were housed 4 to a cage for at least 2 weeks before experiment. In experiments in which plasma corticosterone levels were determined, the animals were housed individually for 1 hr before sacrifice.

Drugs. Dihydroergosine methane sulphonate (DHESN, "Lek", Ljubljana, Yugoslavia) was dissolved in distilled water and injected intraperitoneally in doses of 10 mg/kg up to 100 mg/kg per day (expressed as the salt) (Manev & Pericic, 1989; Manev et al., 1989; Pericic & Manev, 1989). Control rats received the same amount of saline (1 ml per 100 g body weight), or no treatment.

Immune response. Humoral immune response to sheep red blood cells (SRBC) (Jerne et al., 1963) and delayed hypersensitivity to bovine serum albumin (BSA) (Hennigsen et al., 1984) were used as the models. In short, SRBC ($2x10^9$) were injected intravenously, and 5 days later the number of hemolytic plaque-forming cells (PFC) was determined in the spleen. BSA in complete Freund adjuvant (0.1 ml of the 1:1 mixture, containing 2 mg BSA per ml) was injected subcutaneously; 7 days later the challenging injection of 0.075 ml heat-aggregated 2 per cent BSA in saline was injected into the footpad, and the swelling was measured 24 hrs later in comparison to the contralateral footpad injected with saline.

Stress. The animals were stressed either by restraint on boards by means of adhesive tape (3 hr/day) (Boranic et al., 1989), or by forced swimming (5 min/day, 10°C) (Manev et al., 1989), or electroconvulsions (10 mA/50 Hz, 0.1 sec), each repeated 4 times in the course of 4 days.

In the PFC model of the immune response, the first exposure to stress took place 2 hrs after the injection of SRBC, i.e. the animals were stressed on days 1,2,3,4, and killed 24 hrs after the last (fourth) exposure. In the footpad swelling model, the series of 4 stresses was applied either on days 1,2,3,4 (the first exposure 2 hrs after the BSA injection) or on days 4,5,6,7 (and the challenging injection of BSA was given within 2 hrs of the last stress).

Corticosterone in plasma. Samples of plasma were obtained from trunk blood collected from decapitated animals. Corticosterone was determined by a slight modification of a fluorimetric method (Moncloa et al., 1959; Silber et al., 1958).

Statistics. The results were evaluated by the Student's t-test. PFC counts were additionally checked by the U-test. The level of significance was set at $p \angle 0.05$.

Results

Humoral immunity. Repeated electroconvulsions (Table 1) and restraint (Table 2) caused marginal, statistically not significant stimulation of the PFC response; the stress of repeated forced swimming was without appreciable effect (Table 1). Injection of DHESN stimulated the PFC response, but only in doses of 10 mg/kg and 50 mg/kg, whereas 100 mg/kg caused suppression (Tables 2 and 3). If the injection of DHESN preceded the series of repeated restraints, the stimulatory effect resembled that of DHESN alone, i.e. there was no appreciable synergism of drug treatment and stress (Table 2).

Plasma corticosterone levels were elevated in rats subjected to repeated restraint and forced swimming, but not so in rats receiving electroconvulsions (Tables 1 and 2). Injection of DHESN did not result in measurable change of the corticosterone level and did not modify its

Tab. 1: Plaque-forming cell (PFC) response and plasma corticosterone levels of rats immunized with sheep erythrocytes and stressed daily for 4 days by electroconvulsions or swimming in cold water, starting on the day of immunization (means ± s.e.m.).

Group	Treatment	No. of rats	PFC (x 10^3) per spleen	Corticosterone in plasma (µg/100 ml)
A	None (controls)	8	113.8 ± 13.4	45.90 ± 3.98
B	Electroconvulsions (10 mA/50 Hz, 0.1 sec)	8	192.8 ± 64.8	51.93 ± 3.84
C	Swimming (10ºC, 5 min/day)	8	127.1 ± 23.0	60.21 ± 4.50[a]

[a] Significant difference (p / 0.05) from the control group (A).

Tab. 2: Plaque-forming cell (PFC) response and plasma corticosterone levels of rats immunized with sheep erythrocytes, stressed by repeated restraint and/or treated with dihydroergosine (DHESN) 1 hr after the immunization (means ± s.e.m.).

Group	Treatment*	PFC (x 10^3) per spleen	Corticosterone in plasma (μg/100 ml)
A	Saline injections (controls)	835.5 ± 109.1 (8)	31.02 ± 4.82 (7)
B	Restraint	1,178.4 ± 155.8 (8)	54.78 ± 5.10 (8)
C	DHESN (50 mg/kg)	1,311.6 ± 153.8 (8)	35.96 ± 3.29 (6)
D	DHESN + restraint	1,313.4 ± 172.9 (8)[a]	56.24 ± 3.40 (8)[a,c]

* Restraint (3 hr/day) was applied daily for 4 days, the first one 2 hrs after the immunization. DHESN was injected i.p. 1 hr after the immunization...Rats were killed 24 hrs after the last restraint, i.e. 5 days after the immunization.

a,c Significant difference (p/0.05 or better) from the respective groups (A,C). In parentheses, no. of animals; discrepancies are due to lost samples.

Tab. 3: Plaque-forming cell (PFC) response of rats immunized with sheep erythrocytes and treated with dihydroergosine (DHESN).

Group	Treatment*	No. of rats	PFC (x 10^3) per spleen (means ± s.e.m.)
A	Saline injections (controls)	8	171.2 ± 12.5
	DHESN (mg/kg)		
B	10	8	282.2 ± 41.1[a]
C	50	8	247.1 ± 66.2
D	100	8	106.7 ± 21.2[a]

* The drug was given intraperitoneally 1 hr after the antigen. Rats were killed 4 days later.

[a] Significant difference from the control group (A).

Tab. 4: Delayed hypersensitivity to BSA (footpad swelling) in rats treated with repeated stress, dihydroergosine (DHESN), or both (combined results of three experiments; means ± s.e.m.).

Group	Treatment*	No. of rats	Footpad swelling (mm)
A	None, or saline injection controls	23	1.01 ± 0.05 (23)
B	Restraint (3 hrs/day)	16	0.57 ± 0.09 (16)[a]
C	Swimming (5 min/day, 10^0C)	23	0.59 ± 0.09 (23)[a]
D	Electroconvulsions (10 mA/50 Hz, 0.1 sec)	15	0.79 ± 0.06 (15)[a]
E	Dihydroergosine (50 mg/kg + 3 x 10 mg/kg)	15	0.80 ± 0.08 (15)[a]
F	Dihydroergosine Restraint	7	0.30 ± 0.03 (7)[a,b,e]
G	Dihydroergosine Swimming	7	0.68 ± 0.11 (7)[a]

* The animals were stressed from the 4th to the 7th day after immunization and challenged with antigen immediately after the last stress. DHESN was injected intraperitoneally 1 hr before each exposure to stress - the first dose 50 mg/kg, subsequent ones 10 mg/kg each.

a,b,e Significant difference from the respective group (A,B,E).

response to restraint. Thus, no clear correlation was noted between the corticosterone in plasma and the PFC responses.

Delayed hypersensitivity. In three experiments, the exposure to repeated restraint, forced swimming or electroconvulsions from the 4th to the 7th day after immunization with BSA consistently reduced the footpad swelling in response to the BSA challenge on day 7 (Table 4). The exposure to these forms of stress on days 1 to 4 after immunization did not significantly alter the immune response to BSA (data not shown).

Dihydroergosine (50 mg/kg on the 4th day and 10 mg/kg per day on days 5,6,7 after immunization) suppressed the response to BSA (Table 4). The combination of DHESN with restraint resulted in stronger, apparently synergistic, suppression of the response. This potentiation did not occur in combination with swimming.

Discussion

Thus, exposure to repeated stress in the course of 4 successive days after the immunization caused non-significant stimulation of the humoral immune response (PFC count) and suppressed the delayed hypersensitivity reaction (footpad swelling) of female Wistar rats. Enhancement or suppression of the immune response depend on many variables, including e.g. the mode of stress, its timing with regard to antigen injection, differences in species, strain, age and sex of the experimental animals, etc. (Dantzer & Kelley, 1989; Fox & Newberry, 1984; Monjan, 1981; Solomon et al., 1974). In the male rats used in our previous experiments (Boranic et al., 1989), for example, the PFC response was diminished by repeated restraints rather than slightly enhanced, as in the females. As regards the particular models of immune response employed in this work, the footpad swelling is probably more sensitive to the actual level of the corticosteroids, since their anti-inflammatory action may suppress the inflammatory (non-specific) component of the swelling (see Czlonkowska et al., 1987). Indeed, the footpad swelling was suppressed by the stresses applied on days 4 to 7 after the immunization and preceding the challenging injection of antigen on day 7, and not by stresses applied immediately after the immunization (on days 1 to 4) and terminating 3 days before the challenge on day 7.

There was no correlation between alterations of the PFC immune response and corticosterone levels in plasma at the time of assay. For example, repeated stresses (restraint, swimming) caused significant elevation of plasma corticosterone but had a marginal or no effect on the PFC count, whereas DHESN caused significant stimulation of the PFC response without measurable alteration of the corticosterone level at the time of assay (5 days after the injection of DHESN). Two explanations may be offered: (a) the observed effects were mediated by mechanisms bypassing or complementing the hypothalamo-pituitary-suprarenal axis (Dantzer & Kelley, 1989; Shavit et al., 1985); (b) the immune response was more "inert" than the fluctuations in hormone secretion, and the alterations of the immunocompetent cell populations mediated by corticosterone at a (vulnerable) stage of the immune response compromised the final outcome of the reaction, although by that time the plasma levels of corticosterone may have returned to the normal range (Cheido et al., 1982; Okimura & Nigo, 1986; Okimura et al., 1986 a,b).

The effects of DHESN essentially resembled those of stress: stimulation of the PFC response (in small doses) and suppression of the delayed hypersensitivity reaction. These alterations may have been caused by central actions of the substance, resulting in activation of the hypothalamo-pituitary-suprarenal axis (or of the alternative pathways) via adrenergic, serotoninergic and, possibly, GABAergic mechanisms. An increase in the corticosterone level occurs 1 hr after treatment with DHESN, which returns to the normal range within 48 hrs (Manev & Pericic, 1988). Behavioural effects of DHESN indicate activation of serotoninergic pathways (e.g. the 5-HT syndrome in rats, myoclonus in guinea pigs) (Pericic & Manev, 1988), and serotoninergic activation is known to result in alteration (usually suppression) of the immune response (Boranic et al., 1989; Devoino et al., 1986; Jackson et al., 1986). Another possibility is that DHESN exerted direct effects on the immuno-competent cells via peripheral adrenergic and/or serotoninergic mechanisms, since monoamine neurotransmitters modulate the immune response at the peripheral cell level (Ameisen et al., 1989; Bonnet et al., 1984; Czlonkowska et al., 1987; Hellstrand & Hermodsson, 1987; Manda et al., 1988; Roszman & Brooks, 1985; Sanders & Munson, 1985; Silverman et al., 1985; Sternberg et al., 1986). DHESN has been shown to antagonize noradrenaline at the postsynaptic and extrajunctional alpha-adrenoceptors (Radulovic et al., 1984), and its central serotoninergic effects (Manev & Pericic, 1988; Manev et al., 1989; Pericic & Manev, 1988), as well as the evidence for its 5-HT2 receptor antagonism (Mück-Seler & Pericic, 1989; Pericic, 1989; Pericic & Manev, 1988; Pericic & Mück-Seler, 1990), permit extrapolation to similar or related peripheral actions. As was recently shown by Ameisen et al. (1989), antagonists of 5-HT2R suppress delayed hypersensitivity reaction by interfering with the secretion of lymphokines from sensitized T-cells. Preliminary experience with the effects of DHESN on immune response *in vitro* (to be published) indicate its action on the immunocompetent cells.

The combination of DHESN and stress apparently reinforced their mutual suppressive effect on delayed hypersensitivity, but there was no synergistic increase in the PFC count. It should be noted, however, that the doses and schedules of DHESN application were different in the two models of immune reaction. In the PFC model, the animals received a single dose of DHESN (50 mg/kg) immediately after the injection of antigen - i.e. 5 days before the PFC assay - and in the footpad swelling model 4 injections of DHESN were given (50 mg/kg plus 3 times 10 mg/kg) on days 4,5,6,7 after the immunization - i.e. the last injection was given immediately before the challenge and the footpad swelling assay. Increased secretion of corticosterone, which accompanied the treatment with DHESN as well as the exposure to stress but waned within a couple of days (Manev & Pericic, 1988), may have influenced the footpad swelling, in particular its inflammatory component, more directly than the PFC formation. Indeed, treatment with DHESN and/or the exposure to stress on days 1 to 4 after the immunization did not influence the footpad swelling elicited on day 7. As shown (Manev et al., 1989), joint action of DHESN and stress potentiates their immediate mutual effect on the corticosterone level (measured 1 hr after the treatment), but cancels the delayed effect (after 48 hrs). This mutual interference of DHESN and stress with regard to corticosterone secretion may account for the lack of synergism with regard to the PFC response, since the PFC count in the spleen reflects redistribution of lymphocyte subpopulations that occurred under hormonal influence at a critical stage of the response (Cheido et al., 1982; Okimura et al., 1986). It should also be noted that the total dose of DHESN that caused suppression of the footpad swelling (80 mg/kg) approached the suppressive dose of the drug in the PFC model (100 mg/kg).

In general, attempts at manipulating the effects of stress on the immune response by means of drugs affecting neuroendocrine functions encounter three sets of interconnected factors: (a) neuroendocrine response to stress; (b) feedback influence of the immune response on neuroendocrine mechanisms; (c) dual effects of the drugs - centrally and peripherally.

References

Ameisen, J.-C., Meade R. & Askenase, P.W. (1989). A new interpretation of the involvement of serotonin in delayed-type hypersensitivity. *J. Immunol.* 142:3171-3179.

Balitsky, K.P., Veksler, I.G., Vinnitsky, V.B., Syromyatnikov, A.V. & Shamalko, Y.U.P. (1983). Nervous system and antitumor defense. In: Balitsky, K.P. (Ed.) Naukcva Dumka, Kiev (in Russian).

Besedovsky, H.O., del Rey, A., Sorkin, E. & Dinarello, C.A. (1986). Immunoregulatory feedback between interleukin-1 and glucocorticoid hormones. *Science* 233:652-654.

Blalock, J.E. & Smith, E.M. (1985). A complete regulatory loop between the immune and neuroendocrine systems. *Federation Proc.* 44:108-111.

Bonnet, M., Lespinats, G. & Burtin, C. (1984). Histamine and serotonin suppression of lymphocyte response to phytohemagglutinin and allogeneic cells. *Cell. Immunol.* 83:280-291.

Boranic, M., Pericic, D., Poljak-Blazi, M., Manev, H., Sverko, V., Gabrilovac, J., Marotti T., Radacic, M. & Miljenovic, G. (1989). Immune response of stressed rats treated with drugs affecting serotoninergic and adrenergic transmission. *Biomed. Pharmacother.* (in press).

Cheido, M.A., Idova, G.V. & Devoino L.V. (1982). Effect of haloperidol on distribution of functionally different cells in immunocompetent organs. *B. Exp. Biol. Med.* 94(8):1108-1110 (in Russian).

Cheido, M.A., Idova, G.I., Kadletsova, O. & Devoino, L.V. (1987). Influence of prostaglandin synthesis blockade on the immunosuppressive effect of serotonin and haloperidol. *Farmakol. T.* 50:51-54 (in Russian).

Culman, J., Kvetnansky, R., Torda, T. & Murgas, K. (1980). Serotonin concentration in individual hypothalamic nuclei of rats exposed to acute immonobilization stress. *Neuroscience* 5:1503-1506.

Czlonkowska, A., Jachowicz-Jeszka, J. & Czlonkowski, A. (1987). (^{3}H) Spiperone binding to lymphocyte in extrapyramidal disease and aging. *Brain Behavior. Imm.* 1:197-203.

Dadhich, A.P., Sharma,V.N. & Godhwani, (1980). Effect of restraint stress on immune response and its modification by chlorpromazine, diazepam and pentobarbitone. *Indian J. Exp. Biol.* 18:756-575.

Dantzer, R. & Kelley, K.W. (1989). Stress and immunity: an integrated view of relationships between the brain and the immune system. *Life Sci.* 44:1995-2008.

Devoino,L., Idova, G., Cheido, M., Alperina, E. & Morczova,N. (1986). Moncamines as immunomodulators - importance of suppressors and helpers of the bone marrrow. *Meth. Find. E.* 8:175-181.

Fox, B.H. & Newberry, B.H. (1984). *Impact of psychoendocrine systems in cancer and immunity*. Hogrefe C.J.: Lewiston-New York-Toronto.

Gisler, R.H. (1973). Stress and the hormonal regulation of the immune response in mice. *Psychother. Psychosom.* 23:197-208.

Gisler,R.H., Bussard, A.E., Mazie, J.C. & Hess R,. (1971). Hormonal regulation of the immune response I. Induction of an immune response in vitro with lymphoid cells from mice exposed to acute systemic stress. *Cell Immunol.* 2:634-645.

Glavin,G.B. (1985). Stress and brain noradrenaline. *A Review. Neurosci. Biobehav. Rev.* 9:233-243.

Hellstrand, K. & Hermodsson, S. (1987). Role of serotonin in the regulation of human natural killer cell cytotoxicity. *J. Immunol.* 139:869-875.

Henningsen, G.M., Koller, L.D., Exon, J.H., Talcott, P.A. & Osborne, C.A. (1984). A sensitive delayed-type hypersensitivity model in the rat for assessing in vivo cell-mediated immunity. *J. Immunol. Methods* 70:153-165.

Jackson, J.C., Cross, R.J., Walker, R.F., Markesberry, W.R., Brooks, W.H. & Roszman, T.L. (1985). Influence of serotonin on the immune response. *Immunology* 54:505-512.

Jerne, N.K., Nordin, A.A. & Henry, C. (1963). The agar plaque technique for recognizing antibody-producing cells. In: Amos, B.& Koprowski, H. (Eds.) *Cell bound antibodies*. Wistar Institute Press, Philadelphia, p. 109-115.

Kadlecova, O., Masek, K., Seifert, J. & Petrovicky, P. (1987). The involvement of some brain structures in the effect of immunomodulators. *Ann. NY Acad. Sci.* 496:394-398.

Keller, S.E., Weiss, J.M., Schleifer, S.J., Miller, N.E. & Stein, M. (1983). Stress-induced suppression of immunity in adrenalectomized rats. *Science* 221:1301-1304.

Kuriyama, K., Kanmori, K. & Yoneda, Y. (1983). Functional alterations in central GABA neurons induced by stress. In: Hertz L., Kyamme E., McGeer E.G., Schoustoe, A. (Eds.). *Glutamine, glutamate and GABA in the central nervous system.* Alan R. Liss, New York, p. 559-569.

Laudenslager, M.L. (1983). Coping and immunosuppression: inescapable but not escapable shock suppresses lymphocyte proliferation. *Science* 221:568-570.

Lenox, R.H., Kant, G.H., Sessions, G.R., Pennington, L.L., Mougey, E.H. & Meyerhoff, J.L. (1980). Specific hormonal and neurochemical responses to different stressors. *Neuroendocrinology* 30:300-308.

Manda, T., Nishigaki, F., Mori,J. & Shimomura, K. (1988). Important role of serotonin in the antitumor effects of recombinant human tumor necrosis factor. *Cancer Res.* 48:5250-4255.

Manev,H. & Pericic, D. (1988). Effect of the potential antidepressant dihydroergosine in rats forced to swim: Influence on plasma corticosterone. *Psychoneuroendocrinology* 6:465- 469.

Manev, H., Pericic, D. & Mück-Seler, D. (1989). Inhibitory influence of dihydroergosine on the aggressiveness of rats and mice. *Pharm. Biochem. Beh.* 32:111-115.

Martindupan,R.C. & Dayer, J.M. (1982). Action of neurotransmitters and psychotrophic drugs on the immune system - mediator role of hormones and clinical implications. *Schw. Med. Wo.* 112:1910-1920.

Moncloa, F., Peron, F.G. & Dorfman, R.I. (1959). The fluorimetric determination of corticosterone in rat adrenal tissue and plasma: effect of administering ACTH subcutaneously. *Endocrinology* 65:717-724.

Monjan, A.A. (1981). Stress and immunologic competence: Studies in animals.In: Ader, R.& Good, R.A. (Eds.) *Psychoneuroimmunology*. Academic Press Inc., New York, p. 185-228.

Mück-Seler, D. & Pericic, D. (1989). Effects of dihydroergosine and imipramine on 5-HT receptors in the rat brain. *Iugoslav. Physiol. Pharmacol. Acta* 25: Suppl. 7, 103-104.

Okimura, T. & Nigo, Y. (1986).. Stress and immune responses 1. Suppression of T-cell function in restraint-stressed mice. *Jpn. J. Pharm.* 40:505-511.

Okimura,T., Ogawa, M. & Yamaguchi, T. (1986). Stress and immune response 3. Effect of restraint stress on delayed-type (DTH) response, natural killer (NK) activity and phagocytosis in mice. *Jpn. J. Pharm.* 41:229-235.

Okimura,., Ogawa, M., Yamaguchi, T. & Sasaki, Y. (1986). Stress and immune response 4. Adrenal involvement in the alteration of antibody response in restraint stressed mice. *Jpn. J. Pharm.* 41:237-245.

Pericic, D. (1989). Imipramine and dihydroergosine possess two components - one stimulating 5-HT_1 and the other inhibiting 5-HT_2 receptors. *Iugoslav. Physiol. Pharmacol.* Acta 25: Suppl. 7, 113-114.

Pericic, D. & Manev, H. (1988). Behavioural evidence for simultaneous dual changes of 5-HT receptor subtypes: Mode of antidepressant action? *Life Sci.* 42:2593-2601.

Pericic,, D. & Manev,H. (1989). Dual species dependent effect of dihydroergosine on the convulsions induced by GABA antagonists. *J. Neural. Transm.* 79.125-129.

Pericic, D. & Mück-Seler, D. (1990). Do imipramine and dihydroergosine possess two components - one stimulating 5-HT_1 and the other inhibiting 5-HT_2 receptors? *Life Sci.* 46:1331-1342.

Pierpaoli,W. & Maestroni, G.J.M. (1978, a). Pharmacological control of the hormonally modulated immune response II. Blockade of antibody production by a combination of drugs acting on neuroendocrine functions. Its prevention by gonadotropins and corticotrophin. *Immunology* 34:419-430.

Pierpaoli,W. & Maestroni, G.J.M. (1978, b). Pharmacologic control of the hormonally modulated immune response III. Prolongation of allogeneic skin graft rejection and prevention of runt disease by a combination of drugs acting on neuroendocrine functions. *J. Immunol.* 120:1600-1603.

Radulovic, S., Djordjevic, N. & Kazic, T. (1984). The effect of ergot alkaloids ergosinine, dihydoergosine and dihydroergotamine on neurotransmission and contractility of the isolated ileum of the guinea pig. *J. Pharm. Pharmacol.* 36:814-819.

Raskova, H., Celeda, L., Lavicky, J., Vanecek, J., Urbanova, Z., Krecek, J., Priborska, Z., Elis, J. & Krejci,I. (1987). Pharmacologic interventions to antagonize stress-induced immune consequences. *Ann. NY Acad. Sci.* 496:436-446.

Rehulka, J. (1988). Effect of repeated stress and administration of phenobarbital on the lymphoid tissue and on protein metabolism in the lymphocytes of infant and adult rats. *Physiol. Bohemosl.* 37:57-65.

Roszman, T.L. & Brooks, W.H. (1985). Neural modulation of immune function. *J. Neuroimmunol.* 10:59-69.

Sanders, V.M. & Munson, A.E. (1985). Norepinephrine and antibody response. *Pharmacol. Rev.* 37:229-248.

Shavit, Y., Terman, G., Martin, F., Levis, J.W., Liebeskind, J.C. & Gale, R.P. (1985). Stress, opioid peptides, the immune system, and cancer. *J. Immunol.* 135:834s-837s.

Silber, R.H., Busch, R.D. & Oslapas, R. (1958). Practical procedure for estimation of corticosterone or hydrocortisone. *Clin. Chem.* 4:278-285.

Silverman, D.H.S., Wu, H. & Karnovsky, M.L. (1985). Muramyl peptides and serotonin interact at specific binding sites and enhance superoxide release. Biochem. *Biophys. Res. Comm.*131:1160-1167.

Sklar, L.S. & Anisman, H. (1981). Stress and cancer. *Psychol. Bull.* 89:369-406.

Solomon, G.F., Amkraut, A.A. & Kasper, P. (1974). Immunity, emotions and stress. With special reference to the mechanisms of stress effects on the immune system. *Ann. Clin. Res.* 6:313-322.

Sternberg, E.M., Trial, J. & Parker, C.W. (1986). Effect of serotonin on murine macrophages: Suppression of Ia expression by serotonin and its reversal by 5-HT_2 serotonergic receptor antagonists. *J. Immunol.* 137:276-828.

Susic, D., Djordjevic, N. & Kentera, D. (1984). Hemodynamic effects of two ergot derivatives in the conscious spontaneously hypertensive rat. *Pharmacology* 29:315-223.

Tuomisto, J., Männistö, P. (1986). Neurotransmitter regulation of anterior pituitary hormones. *Pharmacol. Rev*. 37:249-332.

Walker, R.F. & Codd, E.E. (1985). Neuroimmunomodulatory interactions of norepinephrine and serotonin. *J. Neuroimmunol*. 10:41-58.

Wibran, J. (1985). Enkephalins and endorphins as modifiers of the immune system: present and future. *Federation Proc*. 44:92-94.

Chapter 7

Enhancing the Effect of Acupuncture in Plaque-Forming Cells in Mice

Ryoichi Fujiwara
Zhou gui Tong
Harue Matsuoka
Hideki Shibata
Mitsunori Iwamoto
Mitchel Mitsuo Yokoyama

Department od Immunology
Department of Anesthesiology
Kurume University School of Medicine
Kurume, Japan

Introduction

The therapy of acupuncture was common in oriental traditional medicine for various clinical symptoms, and acupuncture point stimulation (Cheng & Pomeranz, 1979; Pomeranz & Chiu, 1976) is generally known to have anaesthetic or analgesic effects. However, the effect of acupuncture stimulation on immune responses has not been thoroughly investigated; although a little information was gained in the past, the effective mechanism of acupuncture is not yet clearly documented. Previous reports indicate that the effect of acupuncture on the immune response might be due to the release of opioid peptides from the pituitary (Kato et al., 1983).

In our previous studies (Fujiwara & Orita, 1987; Fujiwara et al., 1989), an enhancing effect of pain stimulation on immune responses in mice was documented; it was consequently suggested that the enhanced immune responses following pain stimulation were conceivably due to the activation of helper T-cells. The helper cells were not found in the thymus, but the surface markers of the cells were L3T4$^-$, Lyt-2$^-$ and Thy-1$^+$. The helper T-cells were demonstrated to derive from the bone marrow and to be activated by epinephrine released from the adrenal gland (Fujiwara et al., 1988). Furthermore, the results showing an enhanced immune response in PFC production *in vivo* and *in vitro* following acupuncture stimulation were found to resemble those regarding pain stimulation in mice. The phenomena were therefore considered to be based on activation of helper T-cells via neurotransmitters released from the sympathetic nervous system.

Materials and Methods

BALB/c and C57GL/6 male mice, 8 to 10 weeks old, were used throughout the experiments. The mice were obtained from the Shizuoka Agricultural Cooperative Association for Laboratory Animals.

During cell preparation the spleen and thymus of the mice were removed aseptically, the organs finely minced in RPMI 1640 medium, and the cells then passed through no. 150 wire mesh. The bone marrow was pushed out of the femur using a plastic syringe containing phosphate-buffered saline (PBS; pH 7.4). The obtained cells were washed once in PBS and then hemolyzed by adding 0.75% tris-ammonium chloride solution (pH 7.65). The cells were washed three more times and resuspended in RPMI 1640 at a concentration of 1 x 10^7 cells/ml.

The plaque-forming cells (PFC) in the spleen were measured against SRBC. Spleen cells of mice on the fifth day after *in vivo* sensitization with 2 x 10^8 SRBC were used for the PFC test according to the method of Cunningham and Azenberg (Cunningham & Szenberg, 1968). The PFC test was performed after *in vitro* sensitization of the spleen cells of the non-sensitized mice by culturing with SRBC in RPMI 1640. The culture medium was supplemented with 25 mM HEPES, 300 μg/ml L-glutamine, 100 μg/ml penicillin, 100μg/ml streptomycin, 5 x 10^- 5M 2-mercaptoethanol, and 10% fetal bovine serum (FBS). The cell mixtures were cultured for 4 days with the spleen, bone marrow and thymic cells, respectively, of the mice given acupoint stimulation according to a modification of the method of Mishell & Dutton (1967). The cultures were placed in a humidified incubator at 37°C with a constant gas flow (5% CO_2 in air) for 5 days. PFC responses were determined on day 5 using the Cunningham PFC assay.

After acupoint stimulation, the spleen, bone marrow and thymic cells of BALB/c mice were treated with mitomycin C (50 μg/(ml) at 37°C for 30 min and washed three times in RPMI

1640. The mitomycin-treated cells were cultured with normal BALB/c or C57BL/6 spleen cells and SRBC. The cell concentration was equally adjusted to 7.5 x 10^6 cells well prior to use.

Anti-thy 1.2 antibody (Cedarlane Laboratory) was added to the spleen and bone marrow cell suspension (1 x 10^7 cells/ml) to make a 1:1000 dilution of the antibody concentration. The cell and the antibody mixtures were left for 30 min at 4°C, and the cells were resuspended in RPMI 1640 containing rabbit serum complement (Law-Tox-M-RABBIT COMPLEMENT; Cedarlane) at a final concentration of 10%. The cells with the antibody were further incubated at 37°C for 30 min and then washed three times in RPMI 1640. As a control, cells were treated with complement only.

The drugs were dissolved in physiological saline and were administered to the mice either orally or by subcutaneous injection at a dose of 0.1 ml/10g body weight.

As shown in Fig. 1, BALB/c mice were stimulated 15-120 times with a needle inserted at the acupoint of "Zusanli (St.36)" with manipulations of once/sec. In the control group, the needle punctured at the side of the Zusanli under similar conditions to the acupoint stimulation.

The sciatic nerve was denervated under ether anaesthetic by making an incision into the skin and thigh muscle of the left leg. The nerve was then cut off with scissors. As a control, mice received a similar treatment without the nerve incision. After the surgical operation, the mice were kept for 10 days in a cage under the same environmental conditions.

The drugs used were propranolol chloride (Sumitomo Pharmaceutical Co.), phentolamine (Regitine; Chiba-Takeda), procaine (Omnicain; Daiichi), hexamethonium (Methobramine; Yamanouchi) and naloxone (Naloxone hydrochloride; Sigma No. N-7758).

Results

As shown in Fig. 2, acupoint stimulation in mice, consisting of 120 manipulations per day for 4 days, caused a marked increase in PFC production, but in its absence no increase was evident. When the acupoint stimulation was carried out 15 to 120 times an increase in PFC production was found in the mice after over 30 manipulations (Fig. 3). Based on these results, a standard pulse of 45 manipulations was used in the subsequent experiments. Acupoint stimulation caused an increase in PFC production of 70% over the control group. However,

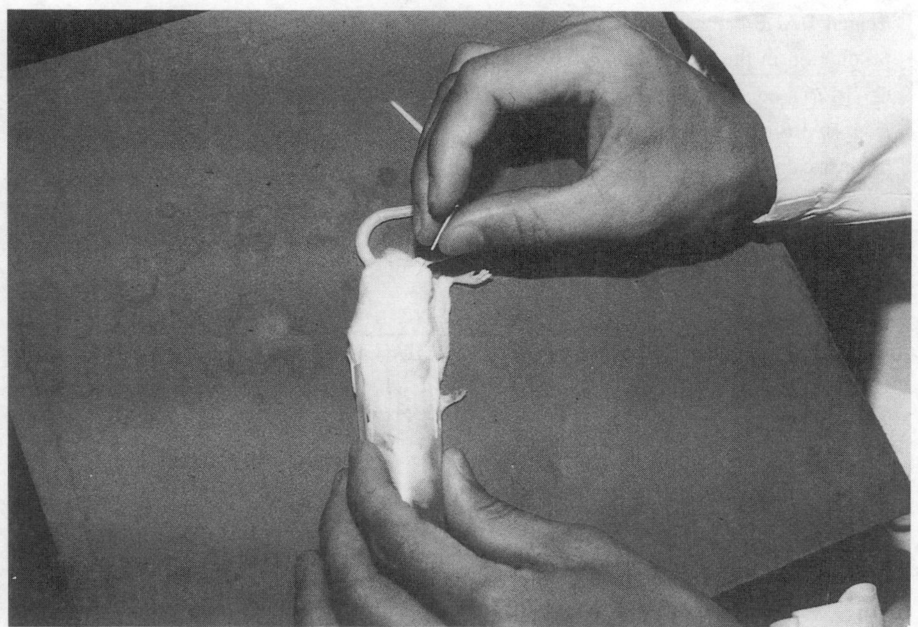

Fig. 1: Photograph of acupuncture point stimulation with a stainless steel needle (0.2 mm in diameter) in the mouse. The needle was inserted into the skin at the approximate depth of the acupoint "Zusanli (St. 36)". Acupoint stimulation was carried out by manipulations once/sec 15-120 times, once a day for 1 to 4 days. The mouse was restrained in the plastic holder in the head forwards position.

this increase was completely blocked by the preadministration of propanolol, 5 ml/kg p.o., while phentlamine, 5 ml/kg p.o., did not affect PFC production after acupoint stimulation (Fig. 4). On the other hand, enhancement of PFC by acupoint stimulation was blocked by pretreatment with hexamethonium, 5 mg/kg s.c., and procain, 5 mg/kg s.c., respectively (Fig. 5). Pretreatment with naloxone injected subcutaneously at a concentration of 0.05 mg/kg also blocked the enhancement of PFC production induced by acupoint stimulation (Fig. 6). PFC production was also blocked upon denervation of the sciatic nerve (Fig. 7).

The effect of acupoint stimulation on helper T-cell activation is shown in Fig. 8. Helper cellswere detected in the spleen and bone marrow cells of mice after acupoint stimulation, but not in the thymic cells. The time required for the onset of helper cell activity induced by acupoint stimulation was two days (45 times/day x 2). The regulatory spleen cells of MMC-treated BALB/c mice given acupoint stimulation also caused a marked increase in PFC production in the spleen cells of BALB/c used as effector cells and in the spleen cells of C57BL/6 used as responder cells (Fig. 9). This helper activity of spleen and bone marrow cells from BALB/c mice was abolished by treatment with anti-thy 1.2 antibody and complement, but not by treatment with complement alone (Fig. 10).

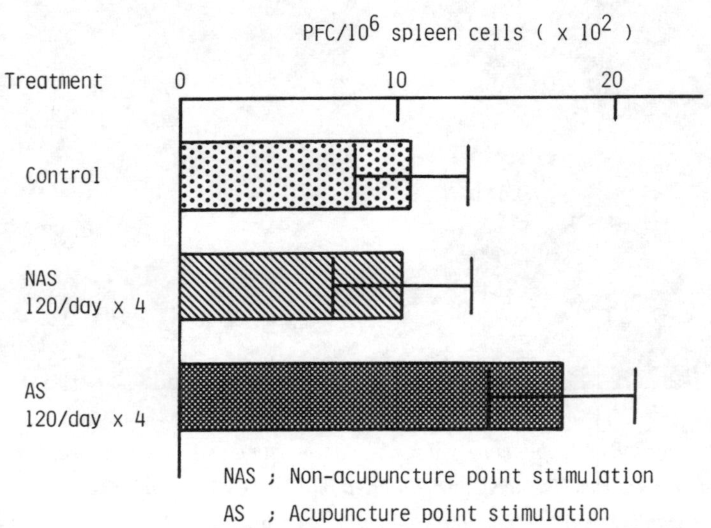

Fig.2: The effect of acupoint stimulation on anti-SRBC PFC production in mice. Mice spleen cells were isolated on day 5 after immunization with 1 x 10^8 SRBC for the in vivo PFC test. Mice were stimulated at the acupoint with a needle for 4 days from day 1 to day 4 after immunization.

Discussion

The present studies reveal that a marked increase in the number of anti-SRBC PFC could be observed after acupoint stimulation. Stimulation caused an increase in the numbers of PFC, but this was blocked by pretreatment with procain and hexamethonium, or by denervation of the sciatic nerve. Furthermore, the number of PFC was also reduced by pretreatment with propranolol and naloxone, although not by phentolamine. These results suggest that the enhancement of PFC in spleen cells induced by acupoint stimulation of SRBC-sensitized mice was due to activation of the sympathetic nervous system through the sensory nervous system

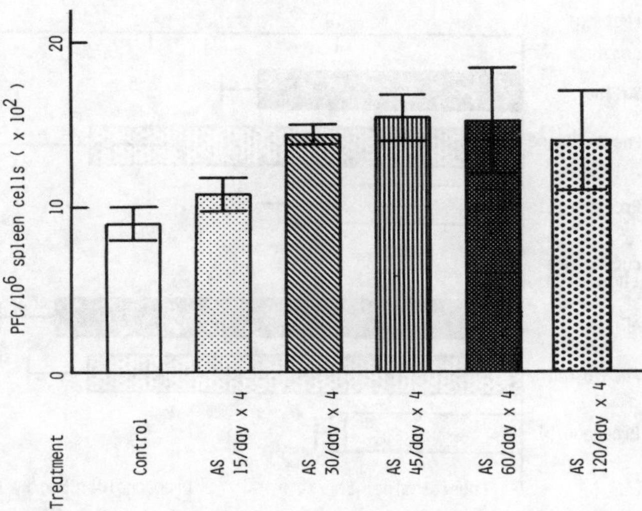

Fig. 3: The influence of the numbers of manipulations during acupuncture point stimulation on PFC production in mice.

following stimulation by acupuncture. Spleen and bone marrow cells of mice not immunized with SRBC mixed with spleen cells of mice stimulated by acupuncture showed an increase in PFC activity, but no increase was detected in the thymic cells. This enhanced PFC activity in spleen and bone marrow cells of normal mice mixed with spleen cells of mice given acupuncture stimulation disappeared upon treatment with anti-thy 1.2 antibody and complement. Thus, the enhancement of PFC induction by acupoint stimulation was attributed to activation of helper T-cells derived from bone marrow, but not from the thymus. Activation of the helper T-cells is considered to occur via neurotransmitters released from the adrenal gland upon stimulation by acupuncture, but not via opiate peptide released from the pituitary. This view is supported by results showing an enhancement of PFC by acupoint stimulation, which was blocked by pretreatment with hexamethonium. Since both propranolol and naloxone blocked the effect of acupuncture on PFC production in mice, the effect of acupuncture may be due to the interaction of epinephrine and opiate peptide released from the adrenal gland (Kurata

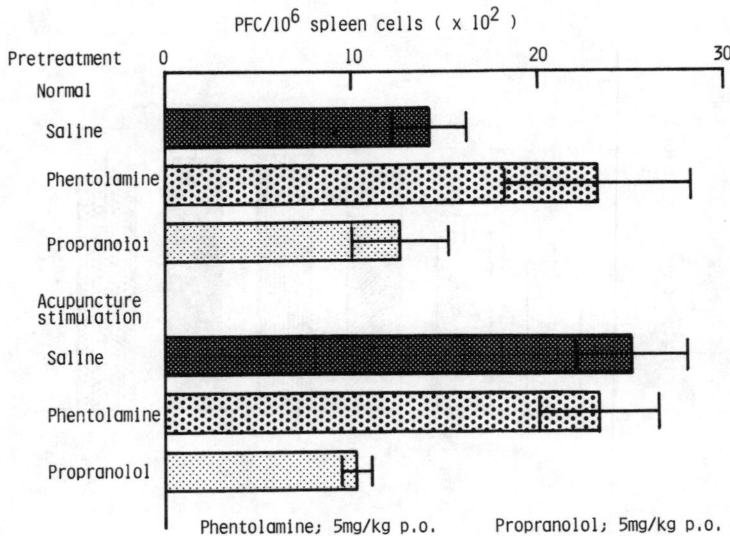

Fig. 4: The effect of phentolamine and propranolol on the enhanced PFC production by acupuncture point stimulation in mice. Phentolamine (5 mg/kg p.o.) and propranolol (5 mg/kg p.o.) were administered 90 min before the stimulation.

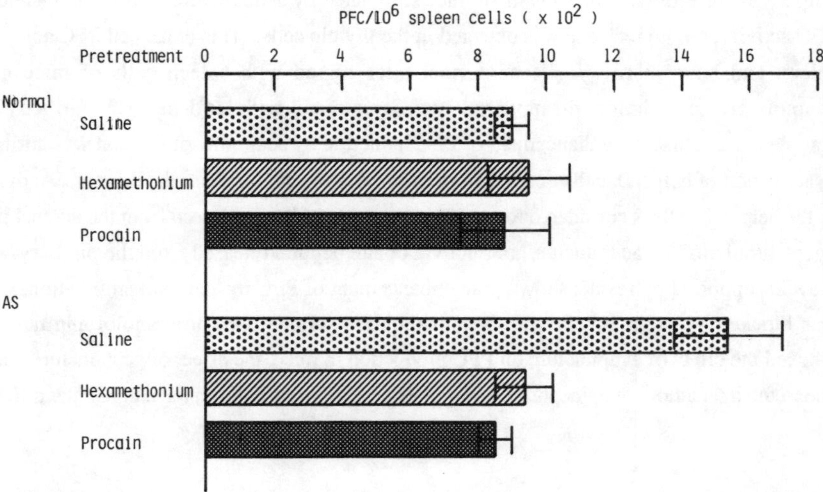

Fig. 5: The effect of the pretreatment with hexamethonium and procain on enhanced PFC production induced by acupuncture point stimulation in mice. Hexamethonium (10 mg/kg s.c.) was administered 60 min and procain (5 mg/kg s.c.) 15 min before the stimulation.

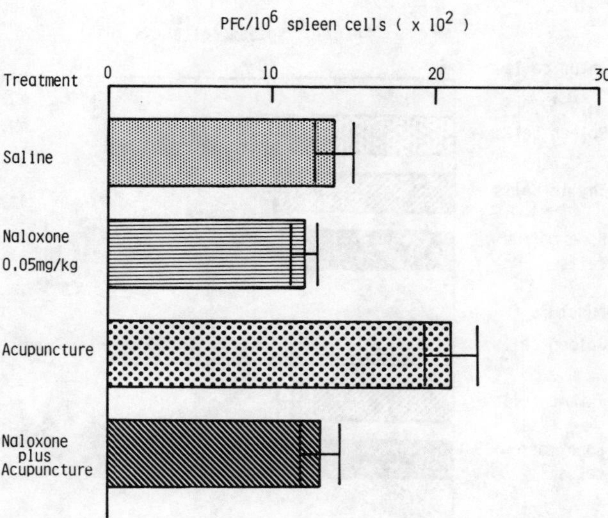

Fig. 6: The effect of naloxone on enhanced PFC production by acupuncture point stimulation in mice. Naloxone (0.05 mg/kg s.c.) was administered 60 min before acupuncture point stimulation.

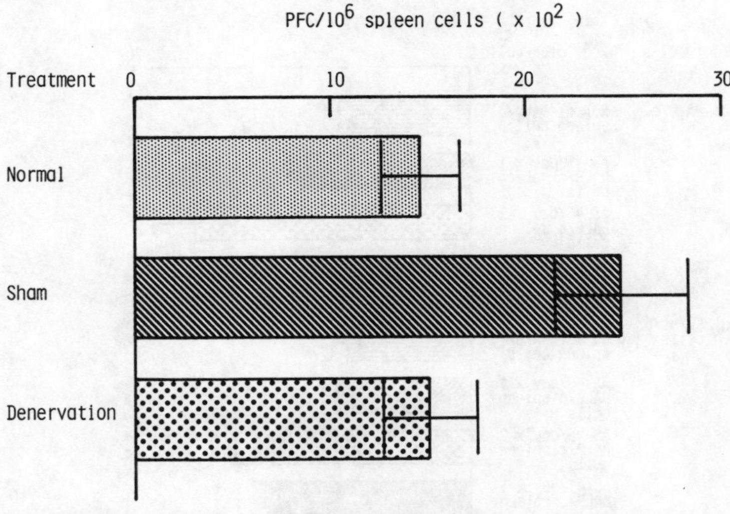

Fig. 7: The effect of denervation of the sciatic nerve on the enhancement of PFC by acupuncture point stimulation in mice. The mice were immunized with SRBC on day 10 after surgery in order to remove the stress. Acupuncture point stimulation was carried out at the acupoint of the left leg.

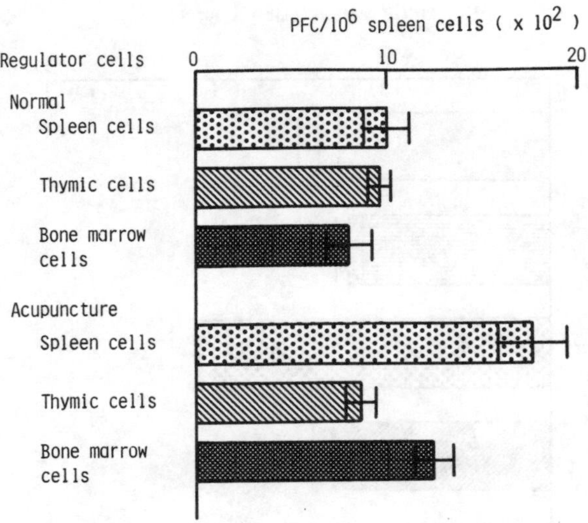

Fig. 8: Enhanced helper cell activity in cells from the spleen and bone marrow from mice given acupuncture point stimulation. Mice were stimulated with needles once a day (45 times/day) for 2 days. Then, spleen and bone marrow cells were used 24 hrs after the second stimulation. The cells were treated with MMC and used as regulatory cells in the in vitro *PFC test.*

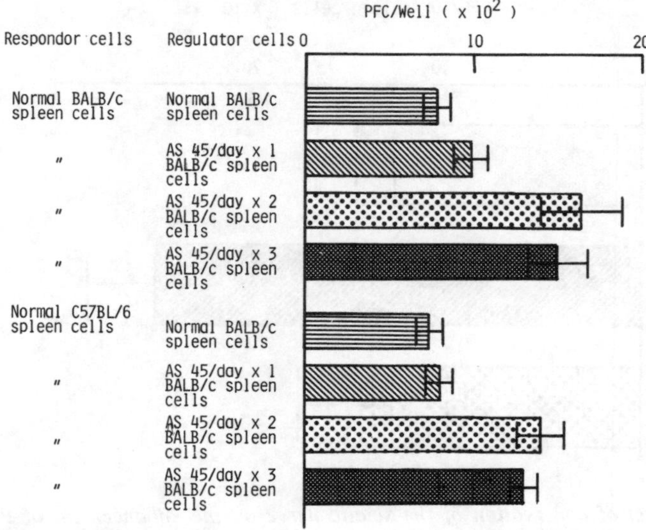

Fig. 9: The kinetics of enhanced helper activity for PFC production by acupuncture point stimulation and H-2 restriction. Mice were given acupuncture point stimulation for 1, 2 and 3 days, and killed 24 hrs after the last stimulation.

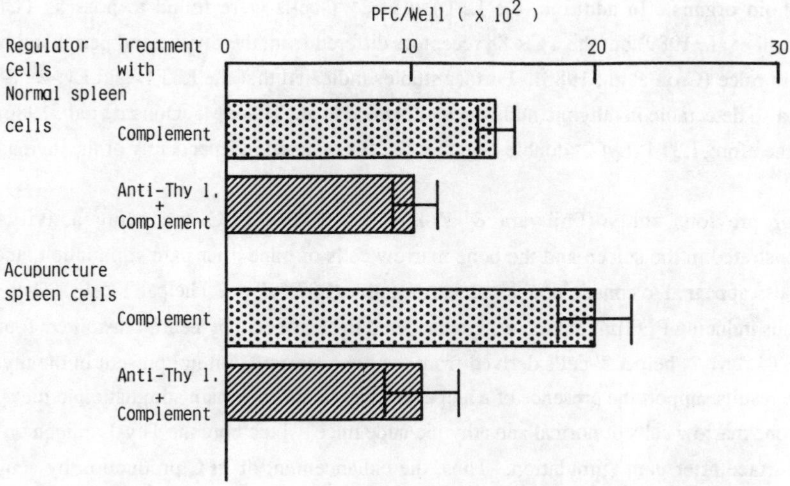

Fig. 10: The influence of anti-Thy 1. 2 antibody and complement on enhanced helper cell activity of spleen cells from mice given acupuncture point stimulation. Mice were given acupuncture point stimulation once a day for 2 days and killed 24 hrs after the second stimulus.

et al., 1989). In our previous study (Fujiwara & Orita, 1987), PFC against SRBC were also enhanced by pain stimulation, similar to acupoint stimulation. In the case of the PFC enhancement by pain stimulation, one stimulus was sufficient for the effect in mice but, in the case of acupuncture, two stimuli were required to induce an enhancement of PFC activity in the spleen cells of mice. Furthermore, our previous study (Kurata et al., 1989) demonstrated that, similar to spleen cells, bone marrow cells are also found to enhance PFC upon in vitro incubation with epinephrine, but not with enkephalin. The enhancing effect of acupuncture on the PFC production is thought to be due to opiate peptide released from the adrenal gland. Furthermore, the spleen cells with PFC enhancing activity induced by acupoint stimulation had the Thy-1 antigen on their cell surface, an antigen which was found in both the spleen and bone marrow cells, but not in the thymic cells. These observations indicated that helper T-cells could be derived from the bone marrow, but independently of the thymus; the cells were also found to differ from L3T4 positive helper T- cells which matured in the thymus.

Recently, attention has been drawn to the existence of a double negative ($L3T4^-/Lyt\text{-}2^-$) T-cell (Bluestone et al., 1987; Ermak & Steger, 1988; Mathieson & Fowlkes, 1984), and such cells were observed in the thymus as immature thymic T-cells. In the latest studies, however, $L3T4^-/Lyt\text{-}2^-$ T-cells were found not only in the thymus but also in the peripheral blood and the lymphoid organs. In addition, the L3T4⁻/Lyt-2⁻ T-cells were found to possess TCR 88 (Takashi et al., 1989) but the TCR 88 receptors differed from the thymic and peripheral blood cells in mice (Cron et al., 1988). Further studies indicated that the L3T4⁻ and Lyt-2⁻ T-cells were also detectable in athymic nude mice (Yoshikai et al., 1986; MacDonald et al., 1986) and that, therefore, L3T4⁻/Lyt-2⁻ double-negative T- cells matured independently of the thymus.

In our previous study (Fujiwara & Yokoyama, 1989), PFC enhancing activity was demonstrated in the spleen and the bone marrow cells of mice after pain stimulation, and the cells also appeared to contain double marker-negative (L3T4⁻/Lyt-2⁻) helper T-cells. Therefore, the cells inducing PFC production were considered to be affected by neurotransmitters found to be L3T4⁻/Lyt-2⁻ helper T-cells derived from the bone marrow, but not present in the thymus. These results support the presence of a helper activity induced by pain stimulation in the spleen and bone marrow cells of normal and athymic nude mice, which bore the Thy-1 antigen on their cell surface after pain stimulation. Thus, the enhancement of PFC production by acupoint stimulation was due to the activation of helper T-cells, which were derived from the bone marrow via neurotransmitters, e.g. epinephrine and/or enkephalin released from the adrenal gland in response to acupoint stimulation.

References

Bluestone, J.A., Pardoll, D., Sharrow, S.O. & Fowlkes, B.J. (1987). Characterization of murine thymocytes with CD3-associated T cell receptor structures. *Nature* 326: 82-84.

Cheng, R.S.S. & Pomeranz, B. (1979). Electro-acupuncture analgesis could be mediated by at least two pain-relieving mechanisms, endorphin and non-endorphin systems. *Life Sci.* 25:1957-1963.

Cron, R.G., Koning, F., Maloy, W., Pardoll, D., Coligan, J.E. & Bluestone, J.A. (1988). Peripheral murine CD3, CD4⁻, CD8⁻, CD8⁻-T lymphocytes express novel T cell receptor structures. *J. Immunol.* 141:1074-1082.

Cunningham, A.J. & Szenberg, A. (1968). Further improvement in the plaque technique for detecting single antibody-forming cells. *Immunology* 14:599-600.

Ermak, T.H. & Steger, H.J. (1988). CD4⁻/CD8⁻ T cells: amplification in spleen of mice following in vivo treatment with monoclonal antibody anti-L3T4. *Eur. J. Immunol.* 18: 231-235.

Fujiwara, R. & Orita, K. (1987). The enhancement of immune response by pain stimulation in mice. 1. the enhancement effect on PFC production via sympathetic nervous system in vivo and in vitro. *J. Immunol.* 138:3699-3703.

Fujiwara, R., Orita, K. & Yokoyama, M.M. (1989). Enhancement of immune response via sympathetic nervous system by pain stimulation in mice. Interactions among central nervous system, neuroendocrine and immune systems. Hadden, J.W., Masek, K. & Nistico, G. (Eds.), pp. 199-208.

Fujiwara, R., Shibata, H. & Yokoyama, M.M. (1988). The characterization of helper T lymphocytes activated by autonomic system. *Proc. Jap. Soc. Immunol.* 18:668.

Fujiwara, R. & Yokoyama, M.M. (1989). L3T4⁻/Lyt-2⁻ double negative helper T cells activated by a sympathetic nervous system. *Proc. Jap. Soc. Immunol.* 19 (in press).

Kato, A., Fujita, H., Shimura, N., Nakamura, C., Hirayama, Y., Kobayashi, A., Ohi, K. (1983). Enhancement of PFC response by acupuncture - endorphin. *Proc. Jap. Soc. Immunol.* 13:744-745.

Kurata, U., Fujiwara, R., Shibata, H., Iwamoto, M. & Yokoyama, M.M. (1989). The effect of neurotransmitter on PFC production in mice. *Proc. Jap. Soc. Immunol.* 19 (in press).

MacDonald, H.R., Blanc, C., Lees, R.K. & Sordat, B. (1986). Abnormal distribution of T cell subsets in athymic mice. *J. Immunol.* 136:4337-4339.

Mathieson, B.J. & Fowlkes, B.J. (1984). Cell surface antigen expression on thymocytes. Development and phenotypic differentiation of intrathymic subsets. *Immun. Rev.* 82:141-163.

Mishell, R.I. & Dutton, R.W. (1967). Immunization of dissociated spleen cells cultured from normal mice. *J. Exp. Med.* 126:423-442.

Pomeranz, B., Chiu, D. (1976). Naloxone blockade of acupuncture analgesia: endorphin implicated. *Life Sci.* 19:1757-1762.

Takashi, T., Steinberg, A.D., June, C.H., &Gause, W.C. (1989). Responsiveness of fetal and adult $CD4^-$, $CD8^-$- thymocytes to T cell activation. *J. Immunol.* 142:2641-2646.

Yoshikai, Y., Reis, M.D. & Mak, T.W. (1986). Athymic mice express a high level of functional chain but greatly reduced levels of T cell receptor messages. *Nature* 324:482-485.

Part III

Psychosocial Factors, Stress and Immunity

Chapter 8

Stressful Events, Depressive Disorders and Immunity

Steven J. Schleifer
Steven E. Keller

University of Medicine and Dentistry
New Jersey Medical School
Department of Psychiatry
New Jersey, U.S.A.

Studies from our laboratory, first at Mount Sinai Medical School in collaboration with Dr. Marvin Stein and more recently at New Jersey Medical School, and others have demonstrated that major stressful life experiences can result in altered immune processes and that similar changes are found in patients with affective disorders. Animal studies demonstrated that a variety of stressors can alter humoral (B-cell) and cell-mediated (T-cell) immunity (Ader, 1981; Monjan & Collector ,1977; Keller et al., 1981; Laudenslager & Ryan, 1983). These studies showed that behavioral and CNS processes can influence several aspects of the immune system and that the effects are related to the nature, duration, and intensity of the stressor as well as to specific characteristics and responses of the stressed organism (e.g. Monjan & Collector, 1977; Keller et al., 1981). Other research has demonstrated influences of higher cortical function on immune processes, including effects related to "coping" and conditioning paradigms (Laudenslager & Ryan, 1983; Ader, 1981).

Animal studies have also begun to elucidate the mechanisms of psychoimmunologic effects and have demonstrated the presence of several if not multiple mediating processes. For example, we investigated the role of the hypothalamic-pituitary-adrenal axis in mediating stress effects on immunity in collaboration with Drs. Jay Weiss and Neal Miller. Using a rat model of unpredictable, unavoidable stress, we found that stress-induced immunomodulation is influenced by both adrenal- and pituitary-dependent and independent mechanisms (Keller et al., 1981, 1983; Keller et al., 1989). These animal studies suggest that psychoimmunologic effects are extensive but complex and point to the need for comprehensive behavioral and immune assessments and caution in generalizing from any single model.

Bereavement and immunity

Research on life stress and immunity in man has identified several conditions in which altered immunity occurs, including conjugal bereavement (Bartrop et al., 1977; Schleifer et al., 1983; Irwin et al., 1987), sleep deprivation (Palmblad et al., 1979), and examination stress (Kiecolt-Glaser et al., 1984; Dorian et al., 1982). The death of a spouse, which has been associated with increased medical mortality (Helsing et al., 1981), was first reported by Bartrop and coworkers (Bartrop, 1981) to be associated with suppressed lymphocyte function. We investigated the effect of bereavement on immunity in a prospective study of spouses of women with advanced breast carcinoma (Schleifer et al., 1983). Several immune system measures were obtained in fifteen men before and after the death of their wives. We found that the number of circulating lymphocytes and T- and B-cells were not significantly altered, however, lymphocyte functional responses to the mitogens phytohemagglutinin (PHA), concanavalin A (ConA), and pokeweed mitogen (PWM), were significantly lower during the first two months post-bereavement compared with pre-bereavement responses. By the end of the post-bereavement year, mitogen responses had returned to pre-bereavement levels for the majority but not all of the subjects. A small subset, including the youngest bereaved men, showed delayed but exaggerated decreases in immunity that persisted for at least a year. Further analyses suggested that lymphocyte mitogen responses for the sample prior to bereavement did not differ from those of age and sex matched controls. This study suggests that major events such as the death of a spouse induce generalized changes in the functional capacity of the lymphocyte.

Major depressive disorder and immunity

Changes in affective state, including the development of depression, could be involved in the effects of bereavement (and other stressors) on immunity. Bereavement is regularly associated with marked changes in mood state and with neurovegetative symptoms that often suggest the presence of a clinical affective disorder (Clayton et al., 1972; Parkes, 1972). Moreover, depression, like bereavement, has been reported to be associated with increased medical mortality (Odegaard, 1952; Avery & Winokur, 1976; Murphy et al., 1987) and with immune-related disorders (Shekelle et al., 1981; Odegaard, 1952; Cappel et al., 1977). In addition, neuroendocrine functions are altered in many depressed patients (Sachar et al., 1980; Carroll et al., 1976; Whybrow & Prange, 1981) and neurohormones and hypothalamic processes have been shown to modulate immune function (reviewed in Stein et al., 1981).

In our initial studies, we found significantly decreased mitogen responses in drug-free hospitalized patients with major depressive disorders (MDD) (Schleifer, Keller et al., 1984) but not in ambulatory MDD patients (Schleifer, Keller et al., 1985). Hospitalized patients with schizophrenia also showed no immune changes (Schleifer, Keller et al., 1985). These observations suggested a specific link between MDD and immunity, however, the psychoimmunologic effects appeared to be restricted to a subgroup of MDD patients. Characteristics that distinguished the first from the second sample included their being hospitalized and more severely depressed, as well as their being older and more predominantly male. All of these factors were investigated in a study of 91 hospitalized and ambulatory unipolar patients with MDD and 91 matched controls (Schleifer et al., 1989). To further elucidate the nature of the immune effects, this study utilized an expanded battery of immune measures. As in all of our studies, all subjects were free of acute and chronic medical disorders associated with alterations in immunity and were not taking drugs known to affect immune function. They had not been treated with antidepressants for at least the preceding three months. There were no significant differences between the entire sample of depressed patients and their controls for any of the immune measures. Significant patient-control differences were revealed, however, when age, sex, severity of depression, and hospitalization were considered. Most striking was that the relationship between age and lymphocyte function for the controls and for the patients was significantly different for each of the mitogens (ConA, PHA, and PWM). A similar difference in age-immune effects between patients and controls was found for the number of T helper (CD4+) cells. The data suggests that, with increasing age in the middle and later years, patients with major depressive disorder have specific concurrent deficits in T4 cells and in lymphocyte function but not in the other aspects of immunity. In contrast, depressed young adults may have increased T4 cells and lymphocyte activity. An additional independent finding was that severity of depressive symptoms, as measured by the Hamilton Depression Scale (Hamilton, 1967), was associated with lower mitogen responses across all ages. Hospitalization status was associated with the number of T4 cells, with inpatients having significantly lower T4 cells.

The findings of our studies with bereaved and depressed populations demonstrate the need to consider a range of demographic, experiential and psychologic variables in psychoimmunologic processes. They suggest that there are several dimensions of psychoimmunologic effects, for example, age-dependent and independent, and that these effects are linked to specific immune parameters. The biological correlates of such effects require investigation. Our findings of adrenal dependent and independent mechanisms of stress effects on immunity in animals (see above) suggest one possible avenue for such research.

Acute and minor stress models

Further studies have been undertaken to clarify the specific psychosocial and biological links between behavior and immunity by investigating lesser and more acute stressors. We had found, for example, no changes in lymphocyte function in patients hospitalized for elective herniorrhaphy (Schleifer et al., 1985; see also Linn & Jensen ,1983). This, together with the preliminary studies described above indicating a lack of lymphocyte functional differences between spouses of cancer patients prior to bereavement and controls, suggests that lymphocyte functional responses may be altered only with severe life stress, possibly only when associated with a depressive state. Further studies by our group at Mount Sinai and then at UMDNJ have extended these observations and suggest that acute stressors may not influence lymphocyte function, but do alter other aspects of immunity.

Our study investigated 21 women whose spouses had been admitted to a coronary critical care unit. No short term effects of the stressor on quantitative or functional lymphocyte measures were apparent when subjects were compared with matched controls. We found evidence, however, that natural killer cell (NK) activity was altered during the first 2 weeks following exposure to the stress.

In another study of 20 family members of trauma victims studied within one week of the traumatic episode, lymphocyte mitogen responses were found not to differ from those of controls, although levels of depression and anxiety were associated with ConA and PWM responsivity (Schleifer et al., 1989, see also below). There was an association between the stressful event and decreased NK activity (Schleifer et al., 1989).

It therefore appears that, in contrast to classical lymphocyte functional responses which may be relatively insensitive to mild or moderate life stress, NK cell function is altered following less intense stressors. Studies by Kiecolt-Glaser and co-workers (1984, 1986) similarly found changes in NK cell activity in medical students taking examinations.

Role of affective states in stress-related immune changes

Other affective states such as anxiety and anger may influence immunity, and preliminary studies from our laboratory suggest that such affective states may be associated with immune changes opposite to those found with depression (Schleifer et al., 1989; Bartlett et al., 1989). In our studies of family members of trauma victims, we found that lymphocyte function, while not associated with exposure to the stressor per se, was related to the affective state of the subjects. Multiple regression analyses showed that depressive symptoms, measured by the Psychiatric Symptom Index (Ilfeld, 1976) were related to decreased ConA responsivity while anxiety symptoms in the same sample were associated with increased mitogen activity.

In another study, we have been investigating the psychoimmunology of otherwise healthy adolescents living in an inner-city with substantial stressful conditions. Initial analyses of psychological, social, and immunologic data for more than 100 adolescents revealed that depressive symptoms were associated with decreased mitogen (ConA and PWM) responses while perceived life stress was linked to increased PWM response (Keller et al., 1989). We also found that adolescents reporting more aggressive behaviors had relatively increased lymphocyte mitogen responses and NK activity (Bartlett et al., 1989).

Conclusion

Taken together, these studies begin to suggest a patttern of psychoimmunologic relationships that emphasize the nature and intensity of stressful conditions, biological characteristics of the individual, and affective states. Extensive and careful studies investigating the range of psychological and immunologic parameters as well as their interactions are required. Such studies would be facilitated by the identification of more fundamental immune "targets" of CNS and behavioral influences, with work in this area currently underway.

References

Ader, R. (1981). *Psychoneuroimmunology.* Academic Press, New York.

Avery, D. & Winokur,G. (1976). Mortality in depressed patients treated with electroconvulsive therapy and antidepressants. *Arch. Gen. Psychiatry* 33:1029-1037.

Bartlett, J.A., Schleifer, S.J., Keller, S.E. & Cranshaw, M.L. (1989). Immune change associated with aggression and depression. *Am. Acad. Child and Adolescent Psychiatry, 36th Annual Mtg (Abstract).*

Bartrop, R.W., Lazarus, L., Luckherst, E. & Kiloh, L.H. (1977). Depressed lymphocyte function after bereavement. *Lancet* 1:834.

Cappel, R., Gregoire, F., Thiry, L. & Sprecher, S. (1978). Antibody and cell mediated immunity to herpes simplex virus in psychotic depression. *J. Clin. Psychiatry* 39:266-268.

Carroll, B.J., Curtis, G.C. & Mendels, J. (1976). Neuroendocrine regulation in depression: II. Discrimination of depressed from nondepressed patients. *Arch. Gen. Psychiatry* 33:1051-1058.

Clayton, P.J., Halikes, J.A. & Maurice, W.L. (1972). The depression of widowhood. Br. J. *Psychiatry* 120:71.

Dorian, B., Garfinkel, G., Brown, G., Shore, A., Gladman, D. & Keystone, E. (1982). Aberrations in lymphocyte subpopulations and function during psychological stress. *Clin. Exp. Immunol.* 50:132-138.

Hamilton, M. (1967). Development of a rating scale for primary depressive illness. *Br. J. Soc. Clin. Psychol.* 6:278-296.

Helsing, K.J., Szklo, M. & Comstock, G.W. (1981). Factors associated with mortality after widowhood. *Am. J. Public Health* 71:802.

Ilfeld Jr., F.W. (1976). Further validation of a psychiatric symptom index in a normal population. *Psycholog. Rep.* 39:1215-1228.

Irwin, M., Daniels, M., Bloom, E.T., Smith, T.L. & Weiner, H. (1987). Life events, depressive symptoms, and immune function. *Am. J. Psychiatry* 144:437-441.

Keller, S.E., Weiss, J.M., Schleifer, S.J., Miller, E. & Stein, M. (1981). Suppression of immunity by stress: Effect of a graded series of stressors on lymphocyte stimulation in the rat. *Science* 213:1397-1400.

Keller, S.E., Weiss, J.M., Schleifer, S.J., Miller, E. & Stein, M. (1983). Stress induced suppression of lymphocyte stimulation in adrenalectomized rats. *Science* 221:1301-1304.

Keller, S.E., Schleifer, S.J., Liotta, A.S., Bond, R.N., Farhoody, N. & Stein, M. (1988). Stress-induced alterations of immunity in hypophysectomized rats. *Proc. Natl. Acad. Sciences* (USA) 85:92-97.

Kiecolt-Glaser, J.K., Garner, W., Speicher, C., Penn, G.M., Holliday, J. & Glaser, R. (1984). Psychosocial modifiers of immunocompetence in medical students. *Psychosom. Med.* 46:7-14.

Kiecolt-Glaser, J.K., Glaser, R., Strain, E.C., Stout, J.C., Tarr, K.L., Holliday, J. & Speicher, C. (1986). Modulation of cellular immunity in medical students. *J. Behav. Med.* 9:5-21.

Kronfol, Z., Silva Jr., J., Greden, J. et al. (1983). Impaired lymphocyte function in depressive illness. *Life Sciences* 33:241-247.

Laudenslager, M.L. & Ryan, S.M. (1983). Coping and immunosuppression: inescapable but not escapable shock suppresses lymphocyte proliferation. *Science* 221:568.

Linn, B.S. & Jensen, J.J. (1983). Age and immune response to a surgical stress. *Arch. Surg.*118:405-409.

Monjan, A.A. & Collector, M.I. (1977). Stress-induced modulation of the immune response. *Science* 196:307.

Murphy, J.M., Monson, R.R., Olivier, D.C., Sobol, A.M. & Leighton, A.H. (1987). Affective disorders and mortality. *Arch. Gen. Psychiatry* 44:473-480.

Odegaard, O. (1952). The excess mortality of the insane. *Acta Psychiatr. Scand.* 27:353-367.

Palmblad, J., Petrini, B., Wasserman, J., Ackerstedt, T. (1979). Lymphocyte and granulocyte reactions during sleep deprivation. *Psychosom. Med.* 41:273-278.

Parkes, C.M. (1972). *Bereavement: studies of grief in adult life.* Internat. Univ. Press, New York .

Sachar, E.J., Hellman, L., Roffwarg, H.P., Halpern, F.S., Fukushima, D.K. & Gallagher, T.F. (1973). Disrupted 24-hour patterns of cortisol secretion in psychotic depression. Arch. *Gen. Psychiatry* 134:493-501.

Schleifer, S.J., Keller,S.E., Camerino, M., Thornton, J.C. & Stein, M. (1983). Suppression of lymphocyte stimulation following bereavement. *JAMA* 250:374.

Schleifer, S.J., Keller, S.E., Meyerson, A.T., Raskin, M.J., Davis, K.L. & Stein, M. (1984). Lymphocyte function in major depressive disorder. *Arch. Gen. Psychiatr.* 41:484-486.

Schleifer, S.J., Keller, S.E., Siris, S.G., Davis, K.L., Stein, M. (1985). Depression and immunity. Lymphocyte function in ambulatory depressed, hospitalized schizophrenic and herniorrhaphy patients. *Arch. Gen. Psychiatry* 42:129.

Schleifer, S.J., Keller, S.E., Bond, R.N., Cohen, J. & Stein, M. (1989). Major depressive disorder and immunity: Role of age, sex, severity and hospitalization. *Arch. Gen. Psychiatry* 46:81-87.

Schleifer, S.J., Keller, S.E., Scott, B.J., Cottrol, C.H. & Vallente, T.J. (1989). Familial traumatic injury and immunity. *American Psychiatric Assoc., New Research,* San Francisco, CA, May 1989 (Abstract).

Shekelle, R.B., Raynor, W.J., Osfeld, A.M., Garron, D., Bieliauskas, L., Liv, S., Maliza, C. & Paul, O. (1982). Psychological depression and 17 year risk of death from cancer. *Psychosom. Med.* 43:117-1022.

Stein, M., Schleifer, S. & Keller, S. (1981). Hypothalamic influences on immune responses. In: Ader, E. (Ed.). *Psychoneuroimmunology.* Academic Press, New York.

Whybrow, P.C. & Prange, A.J. (1981). A hypothesis of thyroid catecholamine receptor interaction. *Arch. Gen. Psychiatry* 38:106-113.

Chapter 9

Psychological Determinants of Immunoglobulins and Complements in Man

Inger M. Endresen
Holger Ursin

Department of Physiological Psychology
University of Bergen, Norway

Introduction

It has now been well established that the T-cell line is subject to direct control by the nervous system. This control is not only evident from the possible innervation of lymph organs but also from numerous demonstrations of relationships between psychological factors and activity and the levels of T-lymphocytes, Natural Killer cells, and monocytes. However, the psychological influence on the immune system does not seem to be restricted to the T-cell line. There is now increasing evidence that also B-cells are subject to such regulation. In this paper, we review our own data on the relationship between psychological factors and immunoglobulins and complements in man.

The advantage of using these immune parameters is that they are readily available from ordinary blood samples, are rather stable, and may be analyzed with simple kits. Therefore, in our search for reliable and biological indicators of stress, we chose these variables at an early stage. However, the results show an amazing and perplexing degree of complexity.

The data to be reported have been collected over several years. Healthy employees from a wide range of professions and work situations were investigated with a standardized "stress battery".

This includes a health survey, blood samples analyzed for immunoglobulins and complements, psychological defense mecahnisms , anxiety scales and a standardized questionnaire for the experience of stress in each job situation. The basic assumption underlying this work is that job stress is mainly due to psychological factors, that these factors depend on the defense mechanisms used by each individual faced with difficulties, and that the level of coping with the situation will show itself both in anxiety scores and in subjective health indicators.

A total of 516 men and 169 women were tested. The men were firemen, process workers, office workers, lifeboat crews, oil platform workers, air pilots, and divers. The office workers were employed in either insurance or industry. The women were office workers in banking or finance, or nurses.

Method

Instruments

Defense. Psychological defense was measured with the "Life Style Index" (LSI) (Plutchik et al., 1979). The test consists of 92 statements which may be answered with "true" or "false". Sum scores were calculated for each of the eight subscales (Denial, Repression, Regression, Compensation, Projection, Displacement, Intellectualization, and Reaction Formation), where high scores indicated high defense.

Anxiety: Disposition to the experience of anxiety was examined with the "Trait Anxiety Inventory" (STAI-TRAIT) (Spielberger et al., 1970). This is a paper and pencil test consisting of 20 claims about how one usually feels. The four alternative responses give a score from one to four for each item, a high score indicating high anxiety.

Job stress. A translated version of "Cooper's Job Stress Questionnaire" was used to examine experience of stress (Cooper, 1981). This comprises 22 questions, and each answer is rated on a six point scale ranging from zero to five.

Immunological tests

Immunoglobulins (Ig)A, G and M, and complement component C3 were quantified by a nephelometric technique using a Behring Laser Nephelometer with automatic equipment. The monospecific antisera were purchased from Behringwerke AG, Marburg/Lahn, Federal Republic of Germany. C4 and CI esterase inhibitor (CI-INH) were quantified by single radial immunodiffusion using commercial plates from Behringwerke AG.

Data analysis

Data analyses were conducted by means of the SPSS-X statistical package (SPSS-X, 1983). Frequencies, Pearson Correlation and Partial Correlation were used. A significance level of $p < 0.05$ was chosen.

Results and statistical analysis

Mean and standard deviation for the immunoglobulins and complement components are shown in Table 1. The levels of the immunoglobulins and complements were all within normal limits. The first finding was that there was a strong correlation between age and the immune factors. For men, IgM and C4 were significantly correlated to age ($p < .01$), for women such correlations were found for IgM, IgA, C3, C4 and C1-INH ($p <. 01$). Therefore, we controlled for age in the correlation analyses. These results are shown in Table 2.The material now shrank to 312 men and 161 women, due to lack of accurate information on age for some of the groups.

The partial correlation analyses show that there are significant correlations between defense mechanisms and IgA, C4 and C1-INH and between anxiety and IgM for men, and between defense and IgG and C4 for women. The correlation coefficients are low for the total samples of men and women. However, when the various subgroups are investigated many of the correlations are much higher. There is an amazing degree of specificity. The patterns of correlation are either distributed at random, or they suggest a rather high degree of specificity between type of occupation and the defense subscales correlating with a particular immunoglobulin.

In the groups composed of lifeboat crew, divers and office workers in industry (all men), we had no information about age. The correlation analyses for these groups - without controlling for age - showed the following results: In the lifeboat crew group, defense had one positive correlation with IgG ($p < .05$) and three negative ones with C1-INH ($p < .05$). For the divers there were two positive correlations between defense and IgA and one with IgG ($p<.05$). The office workers employed in industry had two positive correlations with IgG ($p < .05$).

Tab. 1: Mean and standard deviation for the immunological measures in the different groups.

MEN

	N	IgM		IgG		IgA	
		X	SD	X	SD	X	SD
Lifeboat crew	38	1.36	0.85	11.5	2.2	2.31	0.80
Firemen	88	1.05	0.48	10.8	2.1	2.26	0.92
Process workers	89	1.66	0.96	12.1	2.1	2.50	0.97
Office workers	57	1.64	0.91	12.7	2.5	2.92	1.37
Air pilots	59	1.87	1.50	11.7	3.0	2.58	1.02
Oil-platform	111	1.44	0.94	12.1	1.7	2.71	1.13
Office workers	44	1.92	1.03	12.0	2.3	2.68	1.12
Divers	30	1.96	0.91	12.3	2.7	2.87	1.10
Total group	516	1.55	1.00	11.8	2.3	2.58	1.08

		IgM		IgG		IgA	
		X	SD	X	SD	X	SD
Lifeboat crew	38	0.83	0.15	0.31	0.09	0.35	0.06
Firemen	88	0.86	0.13	0.29	0.09	0.33	0.06
Process workers	89	0.85	0.16	0.36	0.10	0.36	0.07
Office workers	57	1.02	0.21	0.34	0.09	0.37	0.06
Air pilots	59	0.89	0.34	-		-	
Oil-platform	111	0.90	0.21	0.31	0.09	0.38	0.07
Office workers	44	0.90	0.20	0.35	0.14	0.28	0.05
Divers	30	0.89	0.16	-		-	
Total group	516	0.89	0.21	0.32	0.10	0.35	0.07

WOMEN

		IgM		IgG		IgA	
		X	SD	X	SD	X	SD
Nurses	33	2.19	0.85	13.1	1.9	1.96	0.64
Office workers	94	1.79	0.72	12.5	2.4	2.12	1.10
Office workers	42	2.00	0.84	11.9	2.5	2.26	0.84
Total group	169	1.92	0.79	12.4	2.3	2.12	0.96

		C3		C4		Clinh	
		X	SD	X	SD	X	SD
Nurses	33	0.70	0.12	0.28	0.09	0.27	0.05
Office workers	94	0.74	0.13	0.25	0.07	0.27	0.06
Office workers	42	0.86	0.19	0.30	0.09	0.27	0.06
Total group	169	0.76	0.16	0.27	0.08	0.27	0.06

Tab. 2: Partial correlation (controlled for age) between personality and job-stress and immunological measures (N = 312 men, 161 women).

		IgM	IgG	IgA	C3	C4	C1-inh
MEN							
Firemen	Anxiety				.35**		
	Regr.				.28**		
Process workers	Anxiety				-.29**	-.31**	
	Den.		.25*				
	Regr.					-.23*	
	Comp.			-.29**		-.27*	
	Proj.						-.24*
Oil-platform	Reac.		-.21*				
Office workers	Displ.		-.42**				
Total group	Anxiety	-.14*					
	Comp.					-.12*	
	Displ.			-.13*		-.11*	
	Int.			-.11*			-.13*
WOMEN							
Nurses	Stress			.52**			
	Anxiety	-.65**					
	Regr.		.56**	.36*			
	Comp.				-.45**		
	Proj.	-.36*					
	Reac.	-.38*	.48**				
	LSI-sum		.47**				
Office workers	Repr.			-.34*			
	Proj.					.34*	
Total group	Reac.		.16*			.21**	

* $p < 0.05$
** $p < 0.01$ (two-tailed)

Discussion

Throughout all our investigations on the relationships between immunoglobulins, complements and psychological factors, we have found stable relationships between defense mechanisms and immune functions tied to the B-cell line. However, the correlations are very low, although significant, when the total material is analyzed. On the other hand, it is a consistent finding that when we analyze small and homogenous groups, like nurses or teachers, we find strong and significant correlations between specific defense mechanisms and specific changes in immunoglobulins.

These relationships are stable over time (Mykletun et al., 1988); correlations are consistent within one group over periods of two to three years. The lack of consistency in the correlations between groups must, therefore, be attributed to factors other than pure chance. There is a certain possibility that the various professions select different genetic material. Differences in the immune responses and the relationships to personality specific to each occupation could therefore reflect genetic differences. There is some possibility that this is correct since there are specific relationships between personality types and specific endocrine response patterns (Ursin, 1980). However, the most likely explanation is perhaps an interaction between defense mechanisms and the particular job situation. The many different aspects of teaching (Ursin et al., 1984), somatic nursing, and process working may create demands and reinforcement conditions which, in some cases, favour one type of solution, in other cases, different solutions. Use of a particular defense mechanism may be necessary for the somatic nurse and highly inadequate for the bank employee or for the platform worker. We prefer this explanation since our psychological tests do not reveal any profound differences in personality or coping style and coping resources between the various groups of employees. All values treated in this material are well within the normal range for the psychological factors.

Our data suggest that occupational groups that are subjected to workloads and personal challenge over long periods of time may develop particular immunological profiles. At the present time, our data do not permit any conclusion concerning the development of health risks; our material is far too small and should be followed over a long period of time in prospective studies. However, interesting relationships have been found between these indicators and subjective health (Endresen et al., 1989).

We believe that changes in immunoglobulins may reflect a sustained activation state and that the correlations we have found may be used as indicators of stress, if by this is meant a prolonged exposure to a psychological load that might have somatic consequences. With traditional indicators of activation or of stress response the rise and duration times are too short to be useful indicators of the prolonged state of activation which we are interested in as a possible cause of psychosomatic disease and somatic consequences of job stress. However, the pattern in this correlation matrix seems to represent a level of complexity in the interaction between work environment, psychological properties and somatic changes that goes beyond our present mental conception.

References

Cooper ,C.L. (1981). *The stress check.* Prentice Hall, New York.

Endresen, I.M., Ursin, H.& Tønder, O. (Manuscript). Work-related stress, health symptoms and concentrations of immunoglobulins and complements in plasma.

Mykletun, R.J. (1988).Teacher stress, personality, work-load and health.(Report to Rogalands forskning 1988).

Plutchik, R., Kellerman, H. & Conte, H.R. (1979). A structural theory of ego defenses and emotions. In: Izard C. (Ed.) *Emotions in personality and psychopathology.* Plenum Press, New York, pp. 229-257.

Spielberger, C.D., Gorsuch, R.L.& Luschene, R.E. (1970). *STAI Manual for the STATE-TRAIT ANXIETY INVENTORY ("Self-Evaluation Questionnaire")* Consulting Psychologists Press, Inc., Palo Alto.

SPSS-x Users' guide (1983) USA.

Ursin, H. (1980). Personality, activation, and somatic health. A new psychosomatic theory. In: Levine, S. & Ursin, H. (Eds.) *Coping and health.* Plenum Press, New York, pp. 259-279.

Ursin, H., Mykletun, R., Tønder, O., Værnes, R., Relling, G., Isaksen, E. & Murison, R. (1984). Psychological stress-factors and concentrations of immunoglobulins and complement components in humans. *Scand. J. Psychol.* 25:340-347.

Chapter 10

Depression: Role of Corticotropin Releasing Factor in the Reduction of the Natural Killer Cell Activity

Micheal R. Irwin

Department of Psychiatry
University of California, San Diego, U.S.A.

Introductiom

The work in our laboratory has focused upon two primary objectives: 1) to further characterize the relationship between psychological processes and immune function, and 2) to determine the mechanisms by which the central nervous system communicates with immune cells. This review will emphasize both our clinical and preclinical investigations. First, I will discuss our clinical findings that show a reduction of NK activity in both bereaved women and depressed patients. Then, an animal model will be described which has been used to understand how psychological processes such as depression and anxiety might produce changes in immune function. Corticotropin releasing factor has been centrally administered as a neuropeptide probe in the rat to establish the role of the central nervous system in the modulation of NK activity and to further elucidate the underlying outflow pathways likely to mediate communication between the brain and NK cells.

Importance of natural killer cells

Immunologic response against foreign antigens involves the complex interaction between several immune cells such as the T-helper, T-suppressor, and various killer cells (Hood et al.,

1985). While the role of NK cells in host resistance against viral infections and tumor cell growth has not yet been fully determined, substantial evidence in animals supports the hypothesis that NK cells are important in the control of experimental herpes simplex virus (HSV) and cytomegalovirus (CMV) infections (Lotzova & Herbeman, 1986). For example, an enhanced susceptibility to HSV-1 has been found in mice who are selectively depleted of NK activity and receive HSV-1 simultaneously, but not in mice in which NK-cell depletion is postponed 5 days after the virus inoculation (Habu et al., 1984). Likewise, sensitivity to murine CMV infection increases dramatically in the absence of NK cells; whereas, if cells characteristic of NK cells are transferred, resistance to CMV can occur (Bukowski et al., 1985; Bancroft et al., 1981). In humans with disorders such as Chediak-Higashi syndrome (Padgett et al., 1968), X-linked lymphoproliferative syndrome (Sullivan et al., 1980), or chronic fatigue syndrome (Ritz, 1989), positive correlations have been made between sensitivity to viral infections and depressed killer cell functions, although such relationships are not associated with a total loss of killer cells and may merely be coincidental with the underlying disease processes in which other immune abnormalities are also present. However, Biron et al. (1989), described a case in whom an extreme susceptibility to herpes virus infections was associated with a complete and *specific* loss of natural killer cells, killer cell function, and inducible killer cell activity. Together these data support the contention that natural killer cells are an important immunologic defense against certain of the herpes viruses, but probably not against other viruses.

Regulation of natural killer cells

Regulation of cell-mediated immune responses including NK activity involves the secretion of humoral mediators or lymphokines (Dinarello & Mier, 1987). These lymphokines together form a network of regulatory signals which show considerable overlap in patterns of synergism as well as antagonism. For example, the lymphokine interleukin-1 is produced by nearly all immunologic cell types including natural killer cells, T- and B- lymphocytes, brain astrocytes, microglia and macrophages (Dinarello, 1986; Libby et al., 1986; Scala et al., 1984). Interleukin-1 acts mainly as an endogenous adjuvant serving as a co-factor during lymphocyte activation (Dinarello & Mier, 1987), inducing the synthesis of other lymphokines and the activation of resting T-cells (Kay et al., 1984; Shirakawa et al., 1986). A recently discovered property of IL-1 involves its ability to act on natural killers to induce the expression of the IL-2 receptor (Lubinski et al., 1988). The binding of IL-2 by its receptor is a crucial step in the activation of the NK cell, predominantly larger granular lymphocytes, to form lymphokine-activated killers that are able to lyse a wide range of targets in a non-major histocompatability complex restricted manner (Grimm et al., 1982; Kedar & Weiss, 1983; Itoh et al., 1985; Ortaldo et al., 1986). In addition to the role of immune response modifiers in modulating natural killer cell activity, recent evidence demonstrates that the central nervous system also is capable of modulating natural killer cells *in vivo* through either the autonomic nervous system or the neuroendocrine paths.

Adverse life events, depression, and natural killer cell activity

Clinical studies have shown that adverse life events are associated with a decrement in cell-mediated immune function. One of the most severe life events, the death of a spouse (Weiner, 1985), is associated with a suppression of lymphocyte responses to mitogenic stimulation, alterations of T-cell subpopulations, and a reduction of natural killer cell activity. Schleifer and colleagues demonstrated that a suppression of lymphocyte responses to mitogenic stimulation was found in a sample of bereaved men after the death of the spouse as compared to pre-bereavement baseline values (Schleifer et al., 1983). Similar findings of a suppression of lymphocyte responses have been found in a cross-sectional comparison of bereaved men and women versus age- and sex-matched controls (Bartrop et all, 1977). In our investigations of women who are undergoing bereavement, these observations have been extended to other immune parameters such as NK activity and T-cell subpopulations, and the potential role of psychological processes in modulating these immune changes has been addressed (Irwin et al., 1987, a).

In our first study (Irwin et al., 1987), measures of NK activity and T-cell numbers were compared among three groups of women; those whose husbands were dying of lung cancer, those whose husbands had recently died, and women whose husbands were in good health. Women who comprised the study population were free of chronic medical disorders and none were tested during the week after an episode of infectious disease. Current changes in the spousal relationship and other life experiences were assessed using the Social Readjustment Scale (SRS), and severity of depressive symptoms was rated using the Hamilton Depression Rating Scale (HDRS). On the basis of SRS scores, the sample was divided into one of three groups as shown in Fig. 1. Women whose husbands were healthy were more likely to be classified within the low SRS groups; whereas, women who were anticipating or had experienced the death of their spouse were more likely to be found in the moderate or severe SRS group ($x = 33.7$, $df = 4$, $p < .001$). Age was not significantly different between these three groups. Depressive symptoms were significantly ($p < .05$) more severe in the moderate and severe SRS group as compared to those found in the low SRS group.

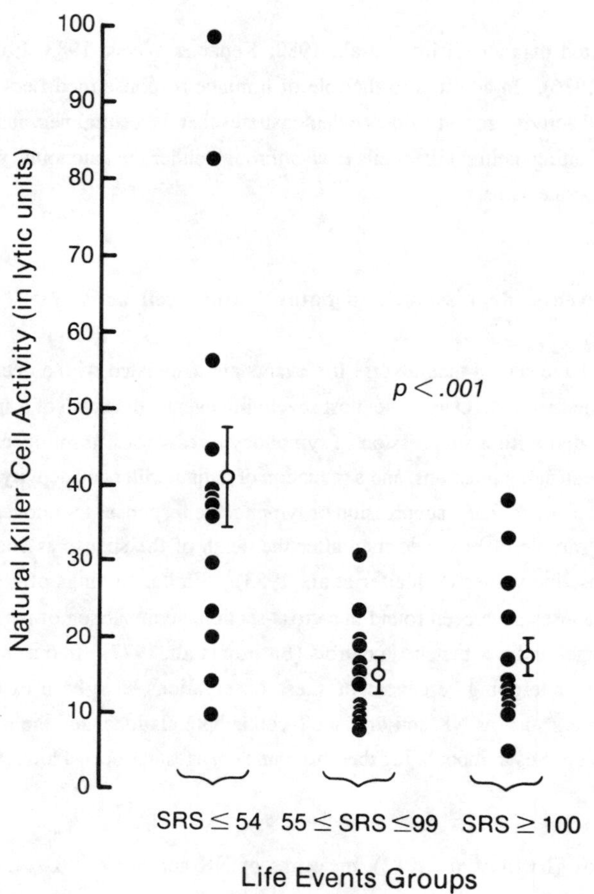

Fig. 1: Natural killer cell activity in women with low, moderate, and high Social Readjustment Rating Scale (SRS) scores. Each point represents the individual's mean of multiple measures.

The immunologic evaluations demonstrated that NK activity expressed in lytic units was significantly ($p < .001$) different between the three groups; the groups with moderate and high SRS scores were found to have significantly ($p < .05$) reduced NK activity as compared to that found in the low SRS subjects (Fig. 1). Neither number of T-helper cells, T-suppressor cells, or the ratio of T-helper to T-suppressor cells were significantly different between the three groups.

Since this cross-sectional data demonstrated that severity of depressive symptoms as measured by the HDRS was significantly correlated with a reduction of natural killer cell activity ($r = .28$,

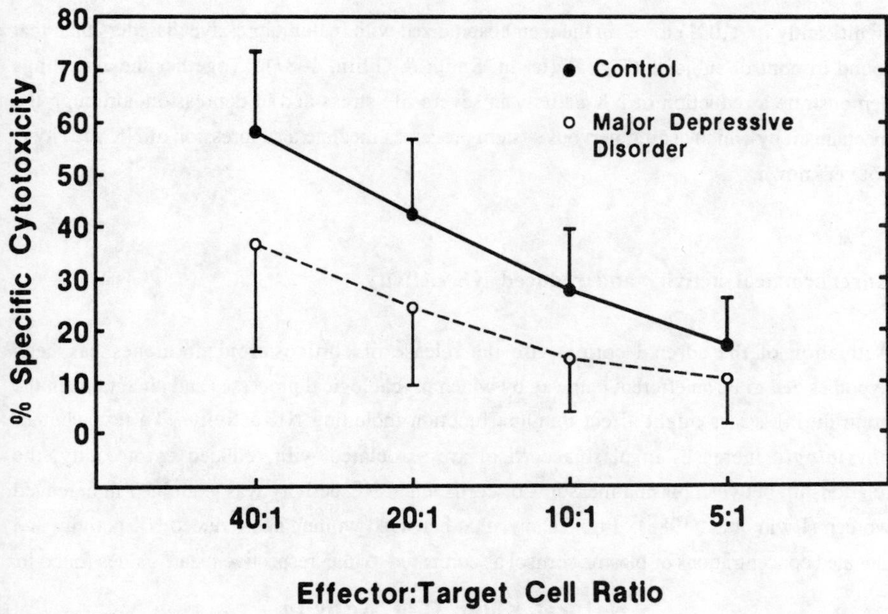

Fig. 2: Natural killer cell cytotoxicity in depressed subjects and controls. Each point represents the mean of the per cent specific cytotoxicity ± SD (n = 19) for each group across the four effector to target cell ratios.

$p < .05$), the potential role of depressive symptoms in mediating these changes of NK activity during bereavement was further evaluated. In a longitudinal design in which a subset of women were followed from pre- to post-bereavement, we examined whether changes in NK activity were related to the actual bereavement event or to changes in severity of the depressive symptoms (Irwin et al., 1987, b). While NK activity did not significantly change in this sample of women from pre- to post-bereavement, differences in the psychological response to the actual death were found between these subjects, and increases in depressive symptoms were correlated ($r = 0.89$, $p < .001$) with a decrease in NK activity from pre- to post-bereavement. Thus, psychological response to the actual death, not merely the death of the spouse is associated with changes in NK activity during bereavement.

Clinical depression and depressive symptoms associated with stressful life events appear to share a common neuroimmunologic alteration (Irwin & Gillin, 1987; Irwin, Smith & Gillin, 1987). For example, in 19 age- and sex-matched pairs comprised of medication-free, acutely depressed patients and control subjects studied on the same day as the patient, NK activity is significantly ($p < .001$) lower in the men hospitalized with major depressive disorders than that found in control subjects (Fig. 2) (Irwin, Smith & Gillin, 1987). Together these findings demonstrate a reduction of NK activity in severe life stress and in depression, although the mechanism by which central nervous system processes mediate a suppression of NK activity is not yet known.

Adrenocortical activity and reduced NK activity

Activation of the adrenal cortex with the release of corticosteroid hormones has been hypothesized to be an efferent pathway by which psychological processes and alterations in the brain during stress might affect immune function including NK activity. To test whether *physiologic* increases in plasma cortisol are associated with reduced cytotoxicity, the relationship between plasma measures of cortisol and NK activity was examined in bereaved women (Irwin et al., 1988). Fig. 3 shows that bereaved women had reduced NK activity and elevated concentrations of plasma cortisol as compared to the respective mean values found in

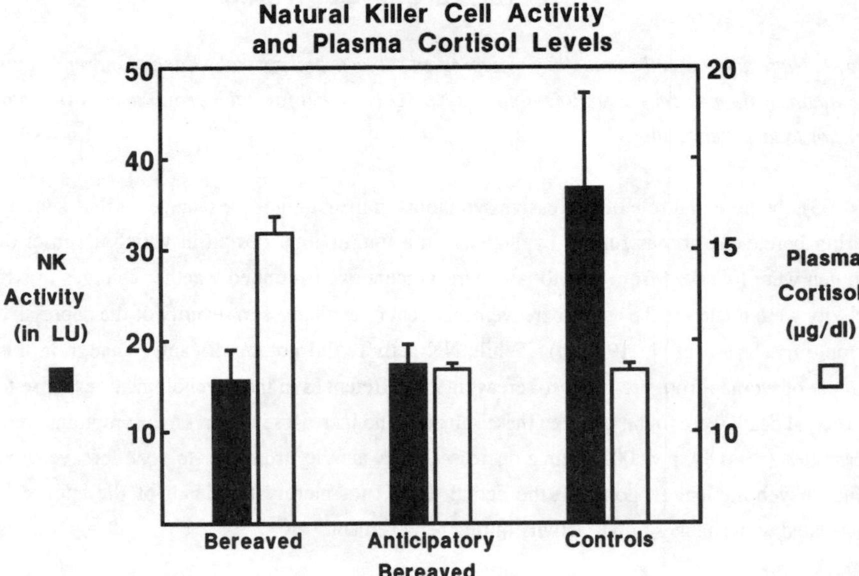

Fig. 3: Natural killer cell activity and plasma cortisol levels in three groups of women: those bereaving the loss of their husbands (n = 9), those anticipating his death (n = 11), and control subjects. Range shown is mean ± SEM of multiple measures of NK activity and plasma cortisol.

the controls. In comparison, anticipatory bereaved subjects had low NK activity, but cortisol levels that were similar to the plasma cortisol mean value of the controls. Plasma cortisol was not significantly correlated with reduced NK activity in the total sample or in any of the three groups. These data, as well as those of other clinical (Kronfol et al., 1986; Kronfol & House, 1985) and preclinical investigation (Keller et al., 1983), suggest that it is unlikely that stress-induced immune suppression is solely mediated by corticosteroid mechanisms and emphasize the need for further studies to clarify the role of the central nervous system in altering immune responses via nervous pathways.

Central modulation of immune function: Action of CRF

Increased concentrations of corticotropin releasing factor have been found in the cerebrospinal fluid of depressed patients (Nemeroff et al., 1984). CRF has been postulated to be a physiological central nervous system regulator that integrates biological responses to stress (Axelrod & Reisine, 1984; Taylor & Fishman, 1988). Thus, CRF is expected to alter not only endocrine function (Vale et al., 1981) but also autonomic (Brown et al., 1982) and visceral functions (Lenz et al., 1987), including immune function (Irwin, Britton & Vale, 1987).

While neuroanatomic studies of the brain have shown that the greatest density of CRF immunoreactive cells and fibers is found in the paraventricular nucleus of the hypothalamus (Paull et al., 1982), immunohistochemical studies have revealed a wide distribution of CRF throughout the brain (Olschowka et al., 1982, a,b; Swanson et al., 1983; Bloom et al., 1982). Furthermore, CRF receptors which are relatively absent in the hypothalamus have been autoradiographically mapped to a number of other extrahypothalamic structures related to the limbic system, and control the autonomic nervous system (DeSouza et al., 1984; Wynn et al., 1984). Thus, in addition to its well established role as a hypothalamic regulator of the pituitary secretion of ACTH and beta-endorphin (Vale et al., 1981), CRF also may act directly in the central nervous system at extrahypothalamic sites. Correspondingly, studies have shown that exogenous CRF administered to animals induces a number of changes in brain function. Intraventricular CRF increases the firing rate of the locus ceruleus (Valentino et al., 1983), activates the autonomic nervous system as reflected by increased plasma concentrations of norepinephrine and epinephrine (Fisher et al., 1982), and produces a pattern of behavioral responses such as decreased feeding and increased locomotor activity (Sutton et al., 1982; Britton et al., 1982; Sherman & Kalin, 1985).

Based upon our interest in understanding the central processes involved in the pathogenesis of immune impairment that is associated with depression, we have examined the role of intraventricular CRF in the regulation of immune function in the rat. Our data demonstrate that central administration of CRF produces a dose-dependent suppression of NK activity which appears specific and independent of direct systemic mechanisms.

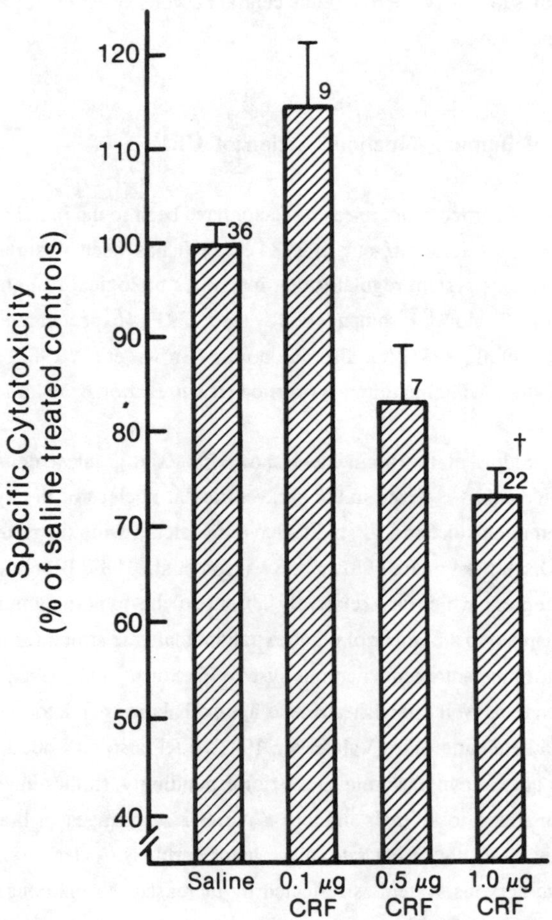

Fig. 4: Effect of central administration of CRF on splenic NK cytotoxic activity (expressed as mean percentage ± SEM of saline-treated controls) (+) significantly ($p < .05$) different from saline group. The number of rats in each group is indicated next to the standard error bars.

Dose response profile of intraventricular CRF: The effect of intraventricular CRF on rat splenic NK activity has been examined using doses of CRF which produce behavioral, pituitary and autonomic actions similar to the responses found in animals subjected to some types of stressors (Irwin, Britton & Vale, 1987). Measurement of NK activity was carried out one hour after intraventricular infusion; a time interval found to result in maximal increases in locomotor activity, plasma norepinephrine and corticosterone levels. In the first study involving the administration of intraventricular CRF, we found a dose-dependent reduction of NK activity across three CRF doses (0.1, 0.5, 1.0 ug) ($F=11.4$, $df = 3.74$; $p < .001$) (Fig. 4). The highest dose of intraventricular CRF (1.0 ug) significantly ($p < .05$) decreased splenic NK activity to $74 \pm 3.1\%$ of the saline-treated group. This finding demonstrated that CRF is capable of modulating immune function *in vivo*, but did not address whether the action of intraventricular CRF was due to a central action of the neuropeptide or a consequence of CRF being distributed from the brain into the peripheral circulation to act directly on lymphocytes.

Lack of direct systemic action of CRF: Additional experiments have tested the possibility that CRF might have a direct peripheral action on NK cells which contributes to the immunosuppressive effect of centrally administered doses. In these experiments, CRF was administered subcutaneously in three doses, 5.0-, 10.0- and 20.0 ug/kg. While it is difficult to equate the dose administered peripherally with that given centrally, the lowest systemic dose of 5.0 ug/kg is roughly equivalent *per rat* to the 1.0 ug ICV-CRF dose, and the 20 ug/kg systemic CRF dose represents about 6.0 ug per rat. Thus, if central CRF (1.0 ug-ICV) is crossing the blood-brain barrier to act peripherally on the natural killer cell, then 5.0 ug/kg CRF administered systemically should have a similar effect. However, as shown clearly in Fig. 5, the 5.0 ug/kg dose of CRF administered subcutaneously had no significant effect upon natural killer cell activity. While there is a trend for NK activity to be reduced following administration of the 20.0 ug/kg dose, this decrease is not statistically significant, and at such a high systemic dose it is possible that CRF crosses the blood-brain barrier from the peripheral circulation and enters the brain. Thus, subcutaneous CRF even in high doses do not appear to alter NK activity significantly.

To examine further the potential effect of CRF on lymphocytes, an additional study was carried out in which rat splenic lymphocytes were incubated for one hour *in vitro* with CRF at a range of concentrations from 10^{-6} M to 10^{-12} M). Throughout the range of CRF concentration, NK activity was similar to the values found in untreated cells, a result demonstrated in three separate experiments. The lack of effect of CRF on NK cells is supported by the lack of CRF binding on purified lymphocyte preparations even though CRF receptors have been identified on monocytes.

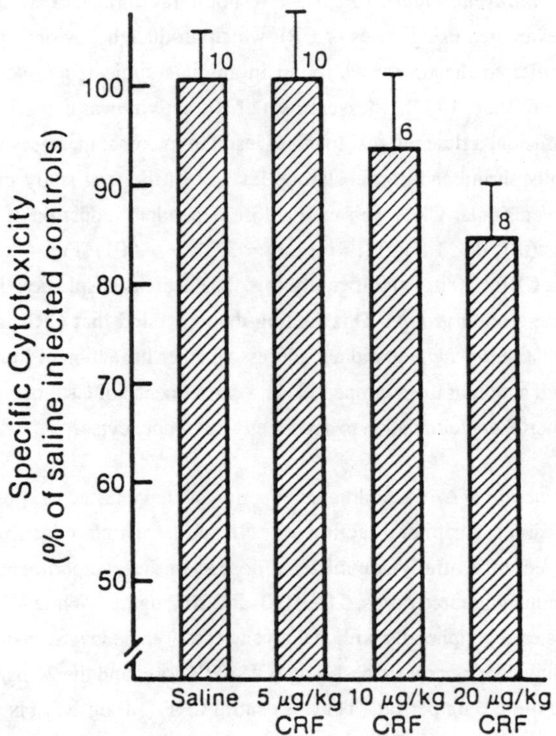

Fig. 5: Effects of systemic administration of CRF at doses of 5, 10, and 20 ug/kg on NK activity (expressed as mean percentage ± SEM of saline-treated controls). Not significantly different between groups (analysis of variance).

These findings indicate that the direct application of CRF does not acutely reduce NK activity and, further, that CRF is unlikely to cross the blood-brain barrier in sufficient doses to alter cytotoxicity. Both of these findings support the hypothesis that the immunosuppressive effect of CRF is centrally mediated and independent of direct systemic mechanisms.

Central specifity of CRF action: The immunosuppressive effect of centrally administered exogenous CRF may be due to the nonspecific effects of the neuropeptide. To address the specificity of this action of CRF, the CRF antagonist alpha-helical was coadministered with CRF. The CRF antagonist was either administered alone or in combination with intraventricular CRF. In another group of rats, the antagonist was injected peripherally followed by a central

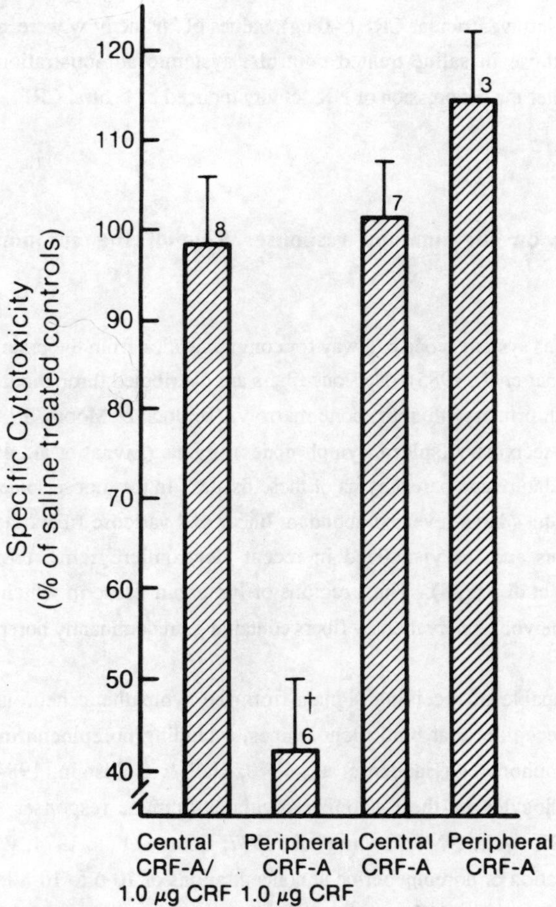

Fig. 6. Central antagonism of the effect of intraventricularly administered CRF on NK cytotoxicity (expressed as mean percentage ± SEM of saline-treated controls). Rats were injected either ICV or systemically with the CRF antagonist immediately before central administration of CRF. The number of rats in each group is indicated next to the vertical standard error bars. NK activity in the systemic CRF antagonist/CRF-treated group was significantly ($p < .05$) lower than that in the saline-, antagonist alone, or central antagonist/CRF-treatment groups.

dose of CRF. Rats coadministered *intraventricular* CRF and the CRF antagonist showed values of NK activity comparable to those observed in saline-treated rats. Thus, central administration of the CRF antagonist significantly attenuated the action of central CRF (Fig. 6).

In contrast, when a *systemic* dose of the antagonist (0.5 mg/kg body weight) was coadministered with intraventricular CRF (1.0 ug), values of NK activity were significantly ($p < .05$) lower than those in saline-treated controls; systemic administration of the CRF antagonist failed to alter the suppression of NK activity induced by central CRF.

Neural influences on the immune response: Role of the autonomic nervous system

The autonomic nervous system is one pathway for communication from the brain to cells of the immune system (Livnat et al., 1985). Nervous fibers are distributed throughout the lymphoid tissues including both primary (thymus, bone marrow) (Bulloch & Moore, 1981; Walcott & McLean, 1985) and secondary (spleen, lymph nodes) organs (Livnat et al., 1985), and are localized in the vasculature and parenchyma of these tissues. In the mouse spleen, fluorescent histochemical techniques have revealed abundant linear and varicose fibers that branch into areas of lymphocytes and, as visualized in recent electromicrograms, terminate on T-lymphocytes (Felten et al., 1988). Thus, regions of lymphoid tissue in which lymphocytes reside receive direct nervous innervation by fibers containing predominantly norepinephrine.

Lymphocytes are capable of receiving signals from the sympathetic neurons innervating lymphoid tissue. Receptors that bind monoamines, including norepinephrine, have been demonstrated on lymphocytes (Hadden et al., 1970; Hall & Goldstein, 1981, 1985), and stimulation of lymphocytes by these agonists regulates immune responses, probably via changes in intracellular cyclic AMP (Strom et al., 1977; Bourne et al., 1974; Watson, 1975). Direct *in vitro* application of norepinephrine at concentrations of 10-6 to 10-8 M reduces NK activity, and this reduction of NK activity following administration of a beta agonist is antagonized by preincubation with a beta antagonist propanolol (Hellstrand et al., 1985). Thus, the concept has emerged that beta adrenoreceptor binding mediates an inhibition of NK activity.

Autonomic nervous system mediation of the CRF suppression: Central administration of CRF produces an acute decrease in splenic NK activity and provides a model to study the relationship between central processes and immune cells via efferent outflow pathways of both the neuroendocrine and the autonomic nervous systems. The role of the autonomic nervous system in mediating CRF-induced suppression of NK cytotoxicity was first explored (Irwin et al., 1988), since central CRF produces an activation of sympathetic outflow, the spleen is extensively innervated by sympathetic fibers, and norepinephrine inhibits NK activity. Using

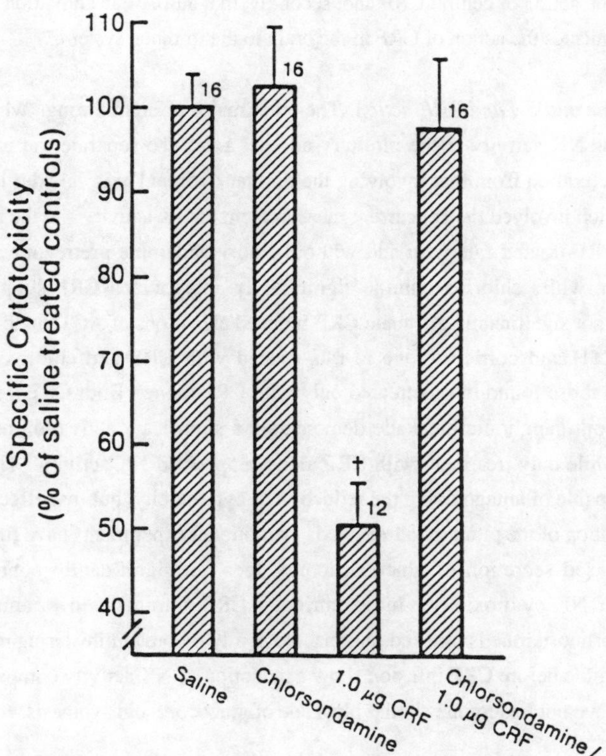

Fig. 7: Effect of ganglionic blockade with chlorisondamine (3 mg/kg IP 60 min before ICV injection) on corticotropin releasing factor (CRF, 1.0 ug ICV)-induced suppression of NK cytotoxicity (expressed as mean per cent ± SE of saline-treated controls). (+) Significantly (p < .001) different from saline group. Number of rats in each group is indicated next to SE bars.

the peripheral ganglionic blocker chlorisondamine, the impact of autonomic activation in directly mediating CRF-induced suppression of NK activity has been examined. Chlorisondamine administered to animals who receive intraventricular CRF significantly antagonized ($p < .05$) CRF-induced elevations of plasma concentrations of norepinephrine and epinephrine, and completely abolished the immunosuppressive effect of CRF on NK activity (Fig. 7). While chlorisondamine given alone produced a modest increase in cytotoxicity as compared to the saline controls, this intrinsic effect of chlorisondamine was not statistically significant. Together these bindings suggest that ganglionic blockade is capable of antagonizing the action of central CRF and, secondly, that autonomic activation is one pathway which communicates the action of CRF in the brain to the immune system.

Neuroendocrine outflow and CRF action: The other major efferent through which CRF might act to suppress NK activity is the pituitary-adrenal axis. To separate the influence of the sympathetic activation from that involving the pituitary-adrenal axis, an additional study was carried out which involved the concurrent measurement of NK activity and the neuroendocrine variables in CRF-treated rats with and without chlorisondamine pretreatment (Irwin et al., 1988). Again, while chlorisondamine significantly antagonized CRF suppression of NK activity, it did not significantly attenuate CRF-induced elevations of ACTH and corticosterone. Levels of ACTH and corticosterone in rats treated with CRF and chlorisondamine were comparable to those found in rats treated only with CRF alone. Both CRF treatment groups with and without ganglionic blockade demonstrate a significant activation of the pituitary-adrenal axis while only treatment with CRF alone suppressed NK activity. Thus, ganglionic blockade is capable of antagonizing the reduction of cytotoxicity, but that effect is dissociated from the activation of the pituitary-adrenal axis. Additional experiments have further suggested that the increased secretion of glucocorticoids does not significantly contribute to CRF suppression of NK cytotoxicity. Intraventricular CRF administered to animals in whom synthesis of corticosterone is blocked pharmacologically by preadministering metyrapone and aminoglutethimide before CRF infusion show a reduction of NK activity comparable to that in animals who have not undergone similar blockade of glucocorticoid synthesis.

These data, evaluating the role of the autonomic nervous system and neuroendocrine systems in mediating the effects of CRF, demonstrate that the autonomic nervous system is a salient efferent pathway by which CRF suppresses NK activity; blockade of this outflow completely antagonizes the action of CRF. Secondly, CRF immunosuppression appears independent of the activation of the pituitary gland. Significant increases in the plasma levels of these hormones can occur without necessarily reducing NK activity.

Acknowledgements

This work was partly supported by NIMH grants #MH44275-01, MH30914, the San Diego VA Clinical Research Center on Alcoholism, and a VA Merit Review.

The work described in "DEPRESSION: ROLE OF CORTICOTROPIN RELEASING FACTOR IN THE REDUCTION OF NATURAL KILLER CELL ACTIVITY" was done as part of our employment with the federal government and is therefore in the public domain.

Parts of this review were previously published.

References

Axelrod, J. & Reisine, T.D. (1984). Stress hormones: their interaction and regulation. *Science:* 224-452.

Bancroft, G.J., Shellam, G.R. & Chalmer, J.E. (1981). Genetic influences on the augmentation of natural killer cells (NK) during murine cytomegalovirus infection: correlation with patterns of resistance. *J. Immunol.* 124:988-994.

Bartrop, R.W., Lazarus, L., Luckherst, E. & Kiloh, L.G. (1977). Depressed lymphocyte function after bereavement. *Lancet* 1:834-836.

Biron, C.A., Byron, K.S. & Sullivan, J.L. (1989). Severe herpes virus infections in an adolescent without natural killer cells. *N. Engl. J. Med.* 320:1732-1735.

Bloom, F.E., Battenberg, E.L. & Rivier, J. et al. (1982). CRF: Immunoreactive neurons and fibers in the rat hypothalamus. *Regul. Pept.* 4:43-48.

Bourne, H.R., Lichtenstein, L.M., Melmon, K., Henney, C.S., Weinstein, Y. & Shearer, G.M. (1974). Modulation of inflammation and immunity by cyclic AMP. *Science* 184:19-28.

Britton, K.T., Koob, G.F. & Rivier, J. (1982). CRF enhanced behavioral effects of novelty. *Life Sci.* 31:363-367.

Brown, M.R., Fisher, L.A. & Spiess, J. et al. (1982). Corticotropin releasing factor: actions on the sympathetic nervous system and metabolism. *Endocrinology* 111:928-931.

Bukowski, J.F., Warner, J.F., Dennert, G. & Welsh, R.M. (1985). Adoptive transfer studies demonstrating the antiviral effect of natural killer cells in vivo. *J. Exp. Med.* 131:1531-1538.

Bulloch, K. & Moore, R.Y. (1981). Innervation of the thymus gland by brainstem and spinal cord in the mouse and rat. *Am. J. Anat.* 162:157-166.

DeSouza, E.B., Perrin, M.H., Insel, T.R., Rivier, C., Vale, W. & Kuhar, M. (1984). CRF receptors in rat forebrain: autoradiographic identification. *Science* 224:1449-1451.

Dinarello, C.A. & Mier, J.W. (1987). Medical intelligence: Current concepts: Lymphokines. *N. Engl. J. Med.* 317 (156):940-945.

Dinarello, C.A. (1986). Interleukin-1: amino acid sequences, multiple biological activities and comparison with tumor necrosis factor (cachectin). *Year Immunol.* 2:68-89.

Felten, S.Y., Felten, D.C., Bellinger, D.C., Carlson, S.L., Ackerman, K.D., Modden, K.S., Olschowka, J.A. & Livnat, S. (1988). Noradrenergic sympathetic innervation of lymphoid organs. *Prog. Allergy* 43:14-36.

Fisher, L.A., Rivier, J., Rivier, C., Spiess, J., Vale, W.W. & Brown, M.R. (1982). CRF: central effects on mean arterial pressure and heart rate in rats. *Endocrinology* 11:2222-2224.

Grimm, E.A, Mazumder, A., Zhang, H.Z. & Rosenberg, S.A. (1982). Lymphokine-activated killer cell phenomenon I. Lysis of natural killer resistant fresh solid tumor cells by interleukin-2 activated autologous human peripheral blood lymphocytes. *J. Exp. Med.* 155:1823.

Habu, S., Akamatsu, K., Tamaoki, N. & Okumura, K. (1984). In vivo significance of NK cells on resistance against virus (HSV-1) infections in mice. *J. Immunol.* 133:2743-2747.

Hadden, J.W., Hadden, E.M. & Middleton, E. (1970). Lymphocyte host transformation I. Demonstration of adrenergic receptors in human peripheral lymphocytes. *J. Cell. Immunol.* 1:583-595.

Hall, N.R. & Goldstein, A.L. (1981). Neurotransmitters and the immune system. In: Ader, R. (Ed.) *Psychoneuroimmunology*. Academic Press, New York, pp. 521-544.

Hall, N.R. & Goldstein, A.L. (1985). Neurotransmitters and host defense. In: Guillemin, R. et al. (Eds.) *Neural modulation of immunity*. Raven Press, New York, pp. 143-154.

Hellstrand, K., Hermodsson, S. & Strannegard, O. (1985). Evidence for a beta-adrenoceptor mediated regulation of human natural killer cells. *J. Immunol.* 134:4095-4099.

Hood, L.E., Weisman, I.L., Wood, H.B. & Wilson, J.H. (1985). *Immunology*. Benjamin Cummings, Menlo Park, CA.

Irwin, M.R., Britton, K.T. & Vale, W. (1987). Central corticotropin releasing factor suppresses natural killer cell activity. *Brain Behav. Immun.* 1:81-87.

Irwin, M., Daniels, M., Bloom, E., Smith, T.L. & Weiner, H. (1987, a). Life events, depressive symptoms and immune function. *Am. J. Psychiatry* 1, 44:437-441.

Irwin, M., Daniels, M., Risch, S.C., Bloom, E. & Weiner, H. (1988). Plasma cortisol and natural killer cell activity during bereavement. *Biol. Psych.* 24:173-178.

Irwin, M.R., Daniels, M., Smith, T.L., Bloom, E. & Weiner, H. (1987, b). Impaired natural killer cell activity during bereavement. *Brain Behav. Immun.* 1:98-104.

Irwin, M.R. & Gillin, J.C. (1987). Impaired natural killer cell activity among depressed patients. *Psychiatry Res.* 20:181-182.

Irwin, M.R., Hauger, R.L., Brown, M.R. & Britton, K.T. (1988). Corticotropin-releasing factor activates the autonomic nervous system and reduces natural cytotoxicity. *Am. J. Physiology Integ. Reg. Mechanisms* 255:R744-747.

Irwin, M., Smith, T.L. & Gillin, J.C. (1987). Reduced natural killer cytotoxicity in depressed patients. *Life Sci.* 41:2127-2133.

Itoh, K., Tilten, B., Kumagai, K. & Balch, C.M. (1985). Leu-ll+ lymphocytes with natural killer activity are precursors of recombinant interleukin-2 induced activated killer cells. *J. Immunol.* 134:802.

Kay, J.S., Gillis, S., Mizel, S.B., Shevach, E.M., Malek, T.R., Dinarello, C.A., Lachman, L.B. & Janeway, C.A. (1984). Growth of cloned helper T cell line induced by a monoclonal antibody specific for the antigen receptor: interleukin-1 is required for the expression of the receptors for interleukin-2. *J. Immunol.* 133:1339.

Kedar, E. & Weiss, D.W. (1983). The in vitro generation of effector lymphocytes and their employment in tumor immunotherapy. *Adv. Cancer Res.* 38:171.

Keller, S., Weiss, J.M., Schleifer, S.J. et al. (1983). Stress induced suppression of immunity in adrenalectomized rats. *Science* 221:1301-1304.

Kronfol, Z. & House, J.D. (1985). Depression, hypothalamic-pituitary adrenocortical activity and lymphocyte function. *Psychopharmacol. Bull* 21:476-478.

Kronfol, Z., Hover, J.D., Silva, J. et al. (1986). Depression, urinary free cortisol excretion, and lymphocyte function. *Br. J. Psychiatry* 148:70-73.

Lenz, H.J., Raedler, A., Greten, H. & Brown, M.R. (1987). CRF initiates biological actions within the brain that are observed in response to stress. *Am. J. Physiol.* 252(IP=2):34-39.

Libby, P., Ordovas, J.M., Birinyi, L.K., Auger, K.R. & Dinarello, C.A. (1986). Inducible interleukin-1 gene expression in human vascular smooth muscle cells. *J. Clin. Invest.* 78:1432-1438.

Livnat, S., Felton, S.J., Carlton, S.L., Bellinger, D.L. & Felton, D.L. (1985). Involvement of peripheral and central catecholamine systems in neural-immuneinteractions. *Neuroimmunology* 10:5-30.

Lotzova, E. & Herbeman, R.B. (1986). *Immunobiology of NK cells II*. CRC Press Inc., Boca Raton, FLa.

Lubinski, J., Fong, T.C., Babbitt, J.T., Ransone, L., Yodoi, J.J. & Bloom, E.T. (1988). Increased binding of IL-2 and increased IL-2 receptor mRNA synthesis are expressed by an NK-like cell line in response to IL-1. *J. Immunol.* 140:1903-1909.

Nemeroff, C.B., Widerlov, E., Bissette, G. et al. (1984). Elevated concentrations of CSF corticotropin-releasing-factor-like immunoreactivity in depressed patients. *Science* 226:1342-1344.

Olschowka, J.A., O'Donohue, T.L., Mueller, G.P. & Jacobowitz, D.M. (1982). The distribution of corticotropin releasing factor-like immunoreactivity neurons in rat brain. *Peptides* 3:995-1015.

Olschowka, J.A., O'Donohue, T.L., Mueller, G.P. et al. (1982). Hypothalamic and extrahypothalamic distribution of CRF-like immunoreaction neurons in the rat brain. *Neuroendocrinology* 35:305-308.

Ortaldo, J.O., Mason, A. & Overton, R. (1986). Lymphokine-activated killer cells. Analysis of progenitors and effectors. *J. Exp. Med.* 165:1193.

Padgett, G.A., Reiquam, C.W., Henson, J.B & Gorham, J.R. (1968). Comparative studies of susceptibility to infection in the Chediak-Higashi syndrome. *J. Pathol. Bacteriol.* 95:509-522.

Paull, W.K., Scholer, J., Arimura, A., Meyers, C.A., Chang, J.K. & Chang, D. (1982). *Peptides I. pp.* 183-191.

Ritz, J. (1989). The role of natural killer cells in immune surveillance. *N. Engl. J. Med.* 320:1748-1749.

Scala, G., Kuang, Y.D., Hall ,R.E., Muchmore, A.V. & Oppenheim, J.J. (1984). Accessory cell function of human B cells. I. Production of both interleukin-1-like-activity and an interleukin-1-inhibitory factor (cachectin). *J. Exp. Med.* 159:1637-1652.

Schleifer, S.J., Keller, S.E., Camerino, M., Thornton, J.C. & Stein, M.M. (1983). Suppression of lymphocyte stimulation following bereavement. *J.A.M.A.* 250:374-377.

Sherman, J.E. & Kalin, N.H. (1985). ICV-CRH potently affects behavior without altering antinociceptive responding. *Life Sci.* 39:433-441.

Shirakawa, F., Tanaka, Y., Eto, S., Suzuki, H., Yodoi, J. & Yamashita, U. (1986). Effect of interleukin-1 on the expression of interleukin-2 receptor (Tac antigen) on human natural killer cells and natural killer-like cell line (YT cells). *J. Immunol.* 137:551.

Strom, T.D., Lundin, A.P. & Carpenter, C.B. (1977). Role of cyclic nucleotides in lymphocytes activation and function. *Prog. Clin. Immunol.* 3:115-153.

Sullivan, J.L., Byron, K.S., Brewster, F.E. & Purtilo, D.T. (1980). Deficient natural killer activity in X-linked lymphoproliferative syndrome. *Science* 210:535-5.

Sutton, R.E., Koob, G.F. & LeMoal, M. et al. (1982). Corticotropin releasing factor produces behavioral activation in rats. *Nature* 297:331-333.

Swanson, L.W., Sawchenko, P.E. & Rivier, J. et al. (1983). The organization of ovine corticotropin releasing factor (CRF). *Neuroendocrinology* 36:165-186.

Taylor, A.I. & Fishman, L.M. (1988). Corticotropin releasing hormone. *N. Engl. J. Med.* 319:213-222.

Vale, W., Spiess, J., Rivier, C. & Rivier, J. (1981). Characterization of a 41-residue ovine hypothalamic peptide that stimulates secretion of corticotropin and beta-endorphin. *Science* 213:1394-1397.

Valentino, R.J., Foote, S.L. & Aston-Jones, G. (1983). CRF activates noradrenergic neurons of the locus coeruleus. *Brain Res.* 270:363-367.

Walcott, B. & McLean, J.R. (1985). Catecholamine containing neurons and lymphoid cells in a lacrimal gland of the pigeon. *Brain Res.*

Watson, J.J. (1975). The influence of intracellular levels of cyclic nucleotides on cell proliferation and the induction of antibody synthesis. *Exp. Med.* 141:97-111.

Weiner, H. (1985). The concept of stress in the light of studies on disasters, unemployment, and loss: a critical review. In: Zales, M.R. (Ed.) *Stress in health and disease*. American College Psychiatry.

Wynn, P.C., Hauger, R.L., Holmes, M.C., Millan, M.A., Catt, K.J. & Aguilera, G. (1984). Brain and pituitary receptors for corticotropin releasing factor's localization and differential regulation after adrenalectomy. *Peptides* 5:1077-1084.

Chapter 11

Stress Induces an Increase in a Subpopulation of Large Peripheral Immunocytes

Karl-Heinz Schulz
Holger Schulz
Andreas Raedler
Bernd Fittschen
Hans Jürgen Lenz
Andreas Messmer
Dirk Zeichner
Margit von Kerekjarto

University Hospital Eppendorf
Hamburg, FRG

Introduction

In numerous studies interactions between the immune and the nervous system were demonstrated (Ader, 1981; Guillemin et al., 1985; Locke et al., 1985; Jankovic et al., 1987). Physical (Simon, 1984; Fitzgerald, 1988) and in particular psychosocial strain, e.g. bereavement (Bartrop et al., 1977 Schleifer et al., 1985), divorce (Kiecolt-Glaser et al., 1987, 1988) and examination stress Kiecolt-Glaser et al., 1984 Baker et al., 1984) have been shown to influence several immune functions, presumably mediated via the nervous and endocrine systems.

In most of these studies results of *in vitro* assays, e.g. mitogen stimulation tests (Bartrop et al., 1977 Schleifer et al., 1985), Natural Killer Cell Activity assays (NKCA; Kiecolt-Glaser et al., 1984) and changes in the distribution of peripheral blood lymphocyte subsets (Baker et al., 1984) were predominantly used as indicators of altered immune functions or alterations within the immune system (see Schulz & Schulz, in press).

The pathophysiological and clinical relevance of these changes, especially of mitogen stimulation tests are not well understood (Golub, 1987 Maier & Laudenslager 1988 Cohen, 1987). More elaborate assays than the NKCA are expensive, time-consuming and an immediate processing of viable cells is necessary. These restrictions do not allow study designs with large sample sizes and multiple measurement points unless appropriate laboratory facilities are available. Consequently, there is a need for immunological parameters which are easier to assess and which reliably reflect an influence of neuroendocrine and psychological processes on the immune system. In order to investigate the underlying mechanisms of such influences it was demonstrated in several animal stress models:

- that a lowered proliferation rate of immunocytes following exposure to various stressors is not dependent on a rise in endogenous cortisol (Keller et al., 1983; Keller et al., 1988);
- that the immunological alteration following stressor exposure is a time-dependent phenomenon (Monjan & Collector, 1977; Jessop et al., 1987; Odio et al., 1986);
- and that psychological rather than physical stressors are possibly crucial determinants in neuroimmunomodulation (Laudenslager et al., 1983; Laudenslager et al., 1988; Fleshner et al., 1988).

According to Maier & Laudenslager (1988) internal replications of findings are rare and in trying to replicate their own results these authors have failed to demonstrate a reproducible effect of psychological stress on immune function using mitogen stimulation assays. With the exception of psychoneuroimmunological conditioning studies (Ader & Cohen, 1985) external replications of stress studies in the field of PNI are missing. Even though there a few studies using the same stress model (examinations, bereavement) different immunological as well as psychological parameters were used and, therefore, the results of these studies are not crossvalidated. Thus replications of results are urgently necessary. For a more detailed discussion see Schulz & Schulz (in press).

Another line of investigation has demonstrated different effects of hormones which are released under stress (e.g. corticotropin-releasing-factor, CRF, prolactin, beta-endorphin, glucocorticoids, catecholamines; Axelrod & Reisine 1984 Taché et al., 1989) on immunological parameters in animal models (Heijnen et al., 1987; Irwin et al., 1987; Irwin et al., 1988; Ovadia et al., 1987) and in humans (Crary et al., 1983a; Crary et al., 1983b; Toennesen et al., 1984).

In our studies we were searching for an immunological *in vivo* parameter which is fast and reliable to determine and thus could be used in studies with larger sample sizes and multiple sample points.

As the starting-point for our interest in the field of psychoneuroimmunology (PNI) we studied the expression of the T9-antigen (transferrin-receptor) on peripheral immunocytes of patients with different autoimmune diseases (multiple sclerosis, antibody-mediated hemophilia, systemic lupus erythematosus, M. Behcet, immunovasculitis, sarcoidosis, colitis, Crohn's disease) and of control subjects (Raedler et al., 1985 a, 1985 b, 1986, 1987). The T9-antigen is expressed on activated peripheral immunocytes and the percentage of T9+ cells is strongly correlated with the expression of the CD25(Tac)-antigen (Raedler et al., 1986), which is the receptor for IL-2 on lymphocytes. In fluorescence-microscopy studies we observed that these activated cells also seemed to be cells of a larger volume. This could be expected because cells going through the cell-cycle increase in volume while in the S-phase. This observation led us to determine both the cell-volume distribution and the percentage of T9+ cells of peripheral blood lymphocytes (PBL). The percentage of a subset of PBL with a larger volume (Large Immunocytes, LI) is correlated with the expression of activation-associated cell surface antigens (T9) in patients with autoimmune diseases (Raedler et al., 1985 c). However, we observed that a higher percentage of LI could also be observed in healthy control subjects while the percentage of T9+ cells remained low in these subjects. We tested the hypothesis that the percentage of LI is related to psychological variance due to perceived stress stated in a visual analogue scale. We found a correlation of $r = .53$ ($N = 21$, $p < .05$) between the percentage of LI and self-rated stress (unpublished data). In order to confirm our preliminary results we tried replications in two different settings (Study 1 and 2), and used an animal model to investigate possible underlying neuroendocrine mechanisms (Study 3). To further characterize LI, phenotypical studies were performed (Study 4).

Immunological methods

Preparation of lymphocites: Samples of 10 ml of peripheral blood were taken and added to 10 ml of 0.9% saline supplemented with 2000 U of heparin. 2.5 ml of "Lymphoprep" (Nyegaard & Co, Oslo, Norway) was overlayered with 5 ml of the diluted blood and centrifuged for 30 min (20°C, 560*g*). The lymphocytes were recovered from the interphase and washed twice with phosphate-buffered saline (PBS, Gibco Laboratories, St. Lawrence, Mass, USA). The pellet was suspended in 10 ml of cell culture medium (RPMI 1640, Gibco) supplemented with 10% fetal calf serum (FCS, Medac, FRG), and cultured for 2 hr at 37°C for removal of monocytes. Nonadherent cells were collected. 1 ml of blood was used in the animal experiment.

Separation of B-cells by panning: After removal of glas-adherent cells the non-adherent cells were layered on petri dishes (ø 5.5 cm, 5 x 10^6 cells/plate) coated with goat-anti-human Ig (4 ml, 25µl/ml, Tago, CA, USA) After incubation for 30 min at room temperature, nonadherent cells were recovered (Wysocki & Sato, 1978).

Phenotypic analysis by fluorescene activated cell sorter (FACS): Monoclonal antibodies directed against the epitopes CD4, CD8, CD25 and the transferrinreceptor (OX26) were used. Rabbit-anti-rat-IgG and IgM were used for detection of B-cells. As second antibodies FITC-coupled (Fab_2)-goat-anti-mouse Ig or goat-anti-rabbit-Ig were used of the subclass appropriate to the monoclonal antibody. 1 x 10^6 non-glass-adherent cells were incubated (30 min, 4°C) with 5 µl of the appropriate antibody under study and 45 µl medium (RPMI 1640, Gibco) supplemented with 10% FCS. After each labelling step cells were thoroughly washed twice in medium (RPMI 1640, Gibco) supplemented with 10% FCS. Cells were measured for fluorescence and small-angle scatter (cell size) with a FACS IV cell-sorter (Becton and Dickinson). The blue laser line (488 nm, 0,2W) was used for excitation. The green fluorescence was measured using the filter combination KP 650 and LP 530 and correlated with the scatter signal in a 4 x 64 channel histogram.

Determination of LI: After preparation of lymphocytes and removal of monocytes by panning non-adherent cells were collected and suspended in culture medium (RPMI 1640, Gibco). Measurement of the cell volume and of lymphocyte number/500 ml was performed using a Coulter Counter, Model ZM and a Coulter Channelyzer C1000. 1 x 10^6 cells were suspended in an electrically conductive medium (20 ml, Isoton II, Coulter Electronics), flow through a small aperture thus causing a voltage drop by increasing the aperture impedance. The resulting pulses were amplified and visualized by means of an oscilloscope. The height of the signal is a function of the cell volume. According to its amplitude, this signal is assigned to 100 discrete channels. In this way a cell-volume-distribution was established until 10,000 cells were counted in the modal channel. The result of this analysis was a cell volume distribution, which is shown in Fig. 5. In order to determine the percentage of large immunocytes - which we termed LI - the percentage of cells with a larger volume than 360 fl (channel 30) was calculated. The peak at channel 15 in this cell size distribution corresponded to a cell volume of 180 fl (and a diameter of 7 µm assuming perfect round cells). In healthy subjects (N = 32) we found a mean percentage of LI of 9.8% (SD = 4.1%; unpublished data).

Study 1: Colonoscopy

In the first study we examined a possible effect of a threatening diagnostic procedure - a colonoscopy - and hypothesized that patients undergoing colonoscopy are in a stressful situation anticipating both the forthcoming procedure and the resulting diagnosis. We expected that patients would be most stressed immediately before colonoscopy.

Design and Methods: Subjects were 18 patients on the waiting list for a colonoscopy (9 female, 9 male; mean age 54 years, SD = 14.6). Only patients without an illness known to modulate immune function were selected to participate (3 patients with hemorrhoids, 4 with benign polyps and 11 without pathological findings confirmed by colonoscopy).
Blood samples were drawn four hours before (t1), immediately before (t2) and one week after the diagnostic procedure (t3). Cortisol was determined by a radioimmunological standard procedure. Anxiety and subjectively perceived stress were assesed with visual analogue scales (VAS). We predicted

- a rise in the percentage of LI from t1 to t2 and expected lower values at t3;
- a higher level of serum cortisol at t2 than values expected according to circadian rhythms.
- Concerning the psychological variables we assumed that patients would be more anxious and more stressed than stated in the VAS.

Statistical comparisons of central tendency were performed by use of the Wilcoxon matched-pairs signed-rank test.

Results and discussion: Fig. 1 shows the LI percentages at the three time points in both groups.The difference in the mean percentage of LI in the patient sample between the two critical assessment points t1 and t2 is significant (t1: M = 25.3%; SD = 8.3% vs. t2: M = 28.7%; SD = 9.7%; $p < .01$). Our main hypothesis was thus confirmed. Baseline levels arealready higher than those of normal healthy subjects (M = 9.8%; SD = 4.1%). These already heightened baseline levels could account for the only slight increase in LI% values from t1 to t2 (ceiling effect). This finding could be explained by the already heightened values of perceived distress at t1 (M = 39.3; SD = 31.7) compared to values one week later (t3: M = 9.4; SD = 7.4; $p < .01$). An increase in VAS-anxiety scores did not reach the level of significance (t1: M = 33.6; SD = 27.7; t2: M = 42.3; SD = 3 3.7; p = .09). As predicted, the decrease in cortisol values from t1 (M = 98mg/ml; SD = 41.9mg/ml) to t2 (M =

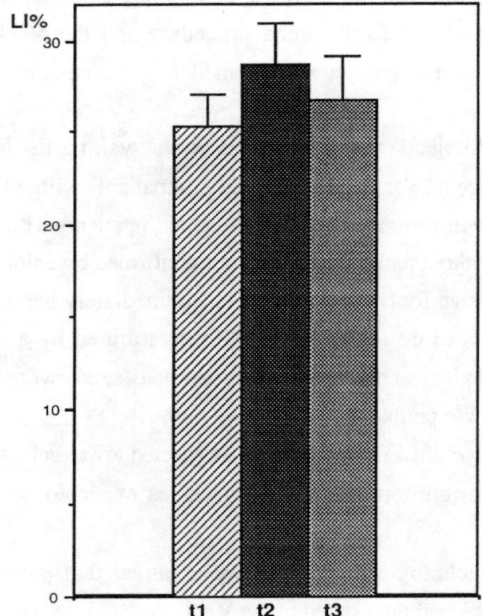

Fig. 1: Mean percentages (+/- SE) of Large Immunocytes (LI%) in the colonoscopy study at the three assessment points.

62.1mg/ml; 34.5mg/ml) was lower than could be expected according to normal values (M = 36.8mg/ml; SD = 15.6mg/ml). Unexpectedly, however, the percentage of LI at t3 remained at the same level as on the day of the diagnostic procedure, which could be due to the endoscopical procedure itself: through microlesions endotoxins could pass into the blood stream causing a modulation of immune function (Kiss et al., 1983 see also Schulz et al., 1989 a, for a more detailed discussion).

Study 2: Examination stress

The second study was carried out with medical students taking part in a major examination. Assuming that students are more stressed just before the exam than one month before we predicted a rise in the percentage of LI during this period.

Sample and design: Medical students taking part in a major examination (N = 61) were randomly selected. Out of 100 students solicited by phone 24 females and 37 males (mean age 23.5 years, SD = 2.8) participated. The most frequent reason for refusal to participate was being out of town at the time of blood drawing. Blood was collected one month (t1) and one or two days (t2) before the examination. To control for the effects of life style and illness on immunological functions, measures of subjectively perceived changes in sleep, nutrition, smoking and alcohol drinking were included as well as reports on clinically apparent illness.

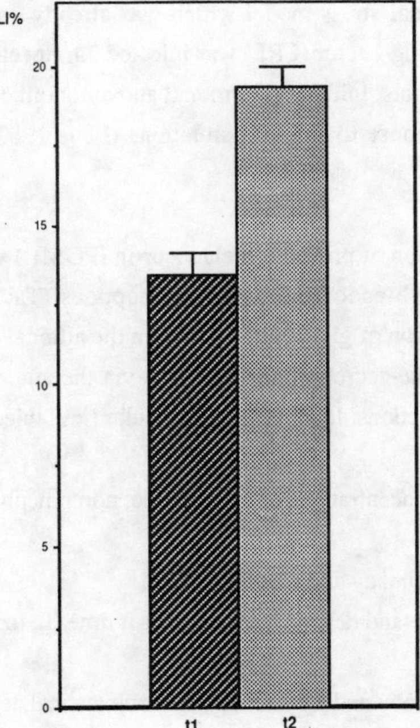

Fig. 2: Mean percentages (+/- SE) of Large Immunocytes (LI%) in the examination stress study at the two assessment points one month (t1) and one or two days (t2) before the examination.

Results and discussion: Fig. 2 shows the mean percentages of LI in Study 2 at one month before or one or two days before the examination.The difference between the means of the two sample points (13.4% vs. 19.3%) is significant (t-test for dependent samples, $t = 7.4$; $df = 60$, $p < .001$). Furthermore, as in Study 1 the percentage of LI at t1 is already heightened compared to values of normal subjects ($M = 9.8\%$; $SD = 4.1\%$). An already high anxiety level at t1 could account for these values. In this study we determined two additional immunological parameters (neopterin and antibodies against herpes simplex virus) and psychological variables concerning anxiety, stress appraisal and coping. These results are described in Fittschen et al. (1989, 1990).

Study 3: Animal experiment

To study possible underlying mechanisms of a rise of LI in peripheral blood following stressor exposure we used an animal stress model which was already established in our departement. Corticotropin-Releasing-Factor (CRF) was injected intrathecally into the third ventricle of male Sprague-Dawley rats, initiating hormonal and autonomic nervous system responses usually observed in response to stressful situations (Lenz 1987 a; Lenz et al., 1987 b).

Release of CRF leads to the excretion of pro-opio-melanocortin (POMC) which is cleaved into adrenocorticotropin (ACTH), b-endorphin and other peptides (Taché et al. 1989). Release of ACTH stimulates secretion of glucocorticoids from the adrenal cortex. CRF not only causes this cascade of hormone-secretion, but also acts via the autonomous nervous system on various physiological functions: Intracerebroventricular (icv) injection of CRF

- significantly increases plasma concentrations of epinephrine, norepinephrine and glucose (hyperglycemia);
- results in a rise in heart beat frequency and blood pressure,
- and inhibits gastric acid secretion and delays intestinal transit time (Lenz et al. 1987 b).

Increased cardiac output, hyperglycemia and a decrease in gastrointestinal activity are typical responses observed in response to stressful events (Selye, 1976. In our experiment we examined whether icv-injection of CRF also results in an increase in the percentage of LI as in the stressful situations described in our studies above.

Sample and design: In short, the experiment was carried out as follows: Using a stereotactical instrument icv-cannulas were placed with their tips inside the third ventricle of male Sprague-Dawley rats (N = 41). After two days rest a catheter was inserted into the right jugular vein. On the day of the experiment, and one day after insertion of the jugular catheter, 2 nmol CRF (experimental group, N = 28) or saline (control group, N = 13) was administered into the cerebrospinal fluid. Blood drawings of 1 ml were obtained before injection of CRF or saline (t0) and six hours later (t1). The correct placement of the cannulas was verified afterwards by histological examination of brain sections . Only animals were included in which correct placement was confirmed.

Results and discussion: The mean percentage of LI in the experimental group rose significantly (Wilcoxon matched-pairs signed-rank test, $p < .001$) from t0 (M = 13.2%, SD = 6.1%) to t1 (M = 22.9%; SD = 7.0%), whereas in the control group the difference was not significant (t0: M = 14.9%; SD = 3.9% vs. t1: M = 13.6%; SD = 7.0%). At t1 the

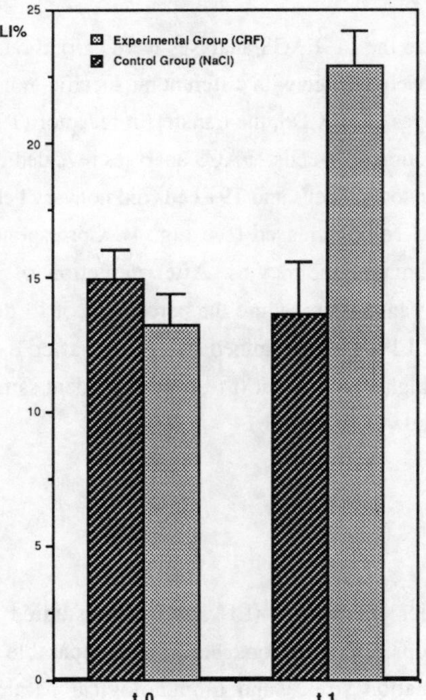

Fig. 3: Mean percentages (+/- SE) of Large Immunocytes (LI%) in the CRF-study at the two assessment points: baseline prior to injection of 2 nmol CRF- or NaCl (t0) and six hours later (t1).

difference between the experimental and control groups was significant (Mann-Whitney-U-Test, $p < .001$; see Fig. 3). Total lymphocyte counts did not differ between the two sample points.

Thus we could demonstrate that intrathecal injection of CRF leads to a pronounced increase in the measured immunological parameter (LI). No difference could be observed after injection of saline, thus the obtained results are not likely to be attributable to effects of the experimental procedure itself. Further analyses concerning dose response and dose time relationship of intrathecal CRF-injection and LI and a comparison of different modes of application (icv vs. iv injection) of CRF have been undertaken (Schulz et al., in preparation).

Study 4: Phenotypical characterization

In order to further characterize the LI, FACS analyses were carried out. Lymphocytes of Sprague-Dawley rats (N = 4) were labeled with different rat-specific monoclonal antibodies (mouse-anti-rat) for the epitopes CD4, CD8, the transferrin-receptor (T9) and with rabbit-anti-rat IgG and IgM for detection of B-cells. FACS analyses revealed that the percentage of helper T-cells, suppressor/cytotoxic cells and T9+ cells did not vary between t0 and t1. In contrast, the percentage of B-cells increased (see Fig. 4). Corresponding results were obtained in studies with human lymphocytes. After depletion of B-cells from the lymphocyte suspension by a panning procedure the percentage of LI decreased (see Fig. 5).In a study of 21 subjects LI were determined before and after B-cell panning; the difference in the means was highly significant (t-test for dependent samples, $t = 5.2$; $df = 20$, $p < .0001$; see Fig. 6; Schulz et al., 1989 b).

Discussion

Changes in an immunological parameter (LI) have been studied in two different psychological stress situations. Interrelations between comparable stress situations (preoperative stress, examination stress) and immunological parameters have been established in several studies (Schulz & Schulz, in press). Irwin et al. (1987, 1988) could demonstrate a decrease in NKCA after using the same animal stress model which was used in our study (intrathecal CRF-injection). This effect could be abolished by pretreatment with the ganglionic blocking agent chlorisondamine which suggests that the observed inhibition of NKCA is due to sympathetic nervous system activity rather than to changes in glucocorticoid levels. Additional evidence for a link between psychological variables and immunological functions is provided by our results. In summary, we could consistently demonstrate a rise in the percentage of large immunocytes (LI) following stressor exposure. This phenomenon was also inducible by intrathecal injection of CRF. Furthermore, it is suggested from preliminary results of our phenotype characterization studies that LI seem to be of the B-cell phenotype.

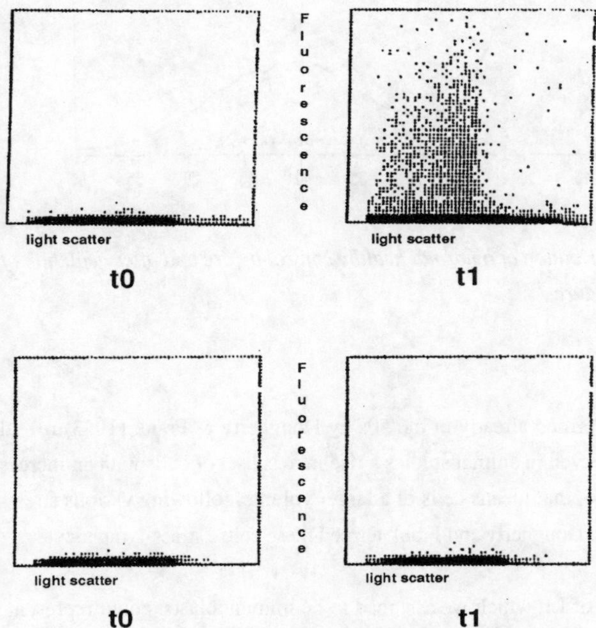

Fig. 4: Results of FACS analysis with rabbit-anti-rat IgG and IgM monoclonal antibodies (first antibody). Upper row: an animal of the experimental group prior to CRF-injection (t0) and six hours later. Lower row: an animal of the control group prior to NaCl-injection (t0) and six hours later.

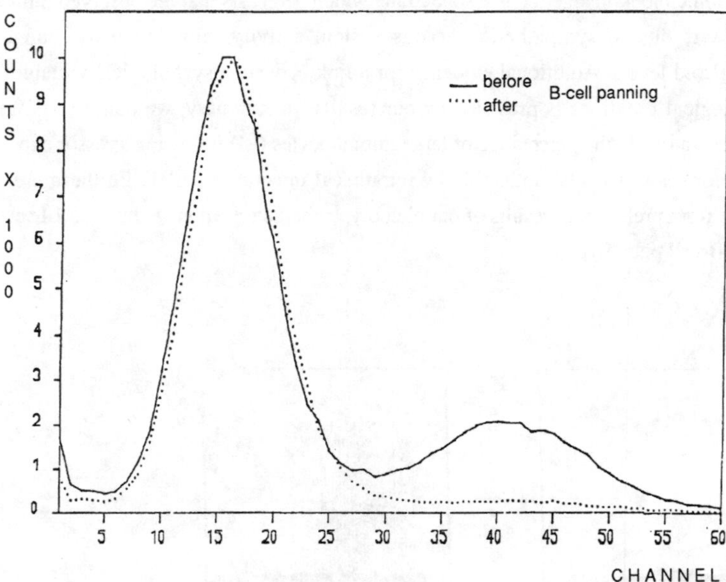

Fig. 5: Cell volume distribution of a normal healthy control before and after depletion of B-cells by a panning procedure.

Experimental work performed already in the 50s by Dougherty & Frank (1953) revealed similar results: they observed in animal studies a rise in a subset of cells with an increased cytoplasmic-nuclear ratio, that means cells of a larger volume, following various stressors or epinephrine injections. Dougherty and Frank termed these cells "stress-lymphocytes".

A rise in the percentage of LI, which we assumed to be immunoblasts, could represent an activation process or could be the result of migration phenomena (Butcher, 1986) induced by physiological changes in stressful situations. A rise in the percentage of LI may represent an enhancement or even a suppression of an overall or some specific immune functions. The possible clinical significance remains to be clarified.

Results of immunological studies favour the hypothesis that migration of lymphocytes is the underlying cause of the phenomenon we observe: It is known that glucocorticoids - in "steroid-resistant" species such as man - lead to a redistribution of lymphocytes (Claman, 1983; Kiess & Hall, 1989). This process seems primarily to affect T-cells, whereas B-cells

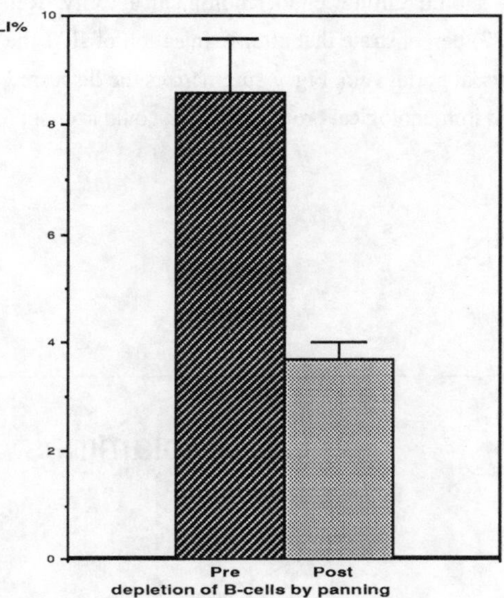

Fig. 6: Percentage of LI (+/- SE) before and after depletion of B-cells by a panning procedure (N=21).

are less affected (Cohen & Crnic 1984). T-cell proliferation induced by mitogens is suppressed or enhanced by b-endorphin, depending on the dosage and the experimental system under study (Gilman et al., 1982; McCain et al., 1982; Heijnen & Ballieux, 1986). ACTH has a synergistic effect on the proliferative signal delivered by either Il-5 (BCGF) or Il-2 to activated B-cells (Alvarez-Mon et al., 1985). Thus ACTH, a hormone which is released in higher amounts in stress situations by the CRF-signal, has an enhancing effect on the proliferation of B-cells, whereas T-cells are redistributed into the tissues and their proliferation could be suppressed. Furthermore, Levitt & Cooper (1987) mention an enhancing effect of glucocorticoids in the process of plasma cell differentiation of activated B-cells. Catecholamines, in addition, have an enhancing or suppressive effect on antibody synthesis by B-cells depending on the time of application (Kishimoto & Ishizaka, 1976; Sanders & Munson, 1985). Proceeding on the assumption of a bidirectional communication between the endocrine and the immune system (Blalock & Smith, 1986), immunological processes, in turn, should initiate endocrinological activity. Related CRF findings of Sapolsky et al. (1987) demonstrate that after iv injection of IL-1 the concentration of CRF rises in the hypophyseal portal vein. Fig. 7 summarizes the discussed interrelations between endocrinological and immunological processes which could account for an increase in LI.

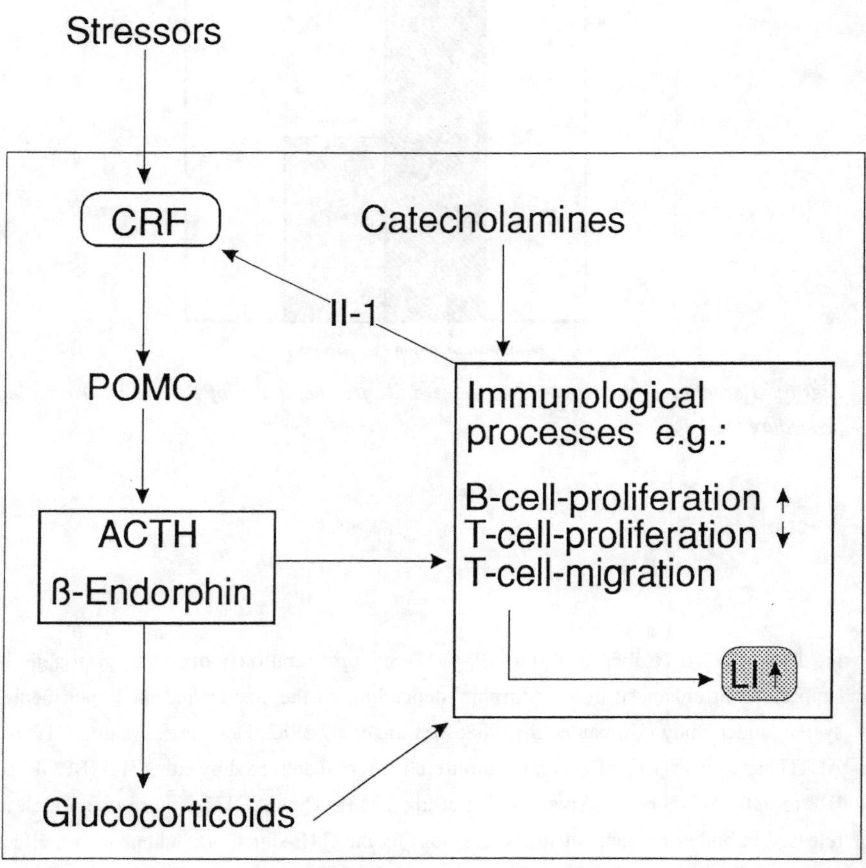

Fig. 7: Some interrelations between endocrinological and immunological processes which could account for an increase in LI (endocrinological feedback-loops not considered, see text).

In summary the two processes described above, i.e. a redistribution of T-cells and a proliferation of B-cells could account for a heightened percentage of LI following stressful situations. Studies to elucidate the physiological significance of this phenomenon are needed.

References

Ader, R. (Ed.) (1981). *Psychoneuroimmunology*. Academic Press, New York.

Ader, R. & Cohen, N. (1985).CNS-immune system interactions: Conditioning phenomena. *Behav. Brain Sci.* 8:379-394.

Alvarez-Mon, M., Kehrl, J.H. & Fauci, A.S. (1985).A potential role for adrenocorticotropin in regulating human B-lymphocyte functions. *J. Immunol.* 135: 3823-3826.

Axelrod, J. & Reisine, T.D. (1984). Stress hormones: Their interaction and regulation. *Science* 224:452-459.

Baker, G.H.B., Byrom, N.A., Irani, M.S., Brewerton, D.A., Hobbs, J.R., Wood, R.J. & Nagvekar, N.M. (1984). Stress, cortisol, and lymphocyte subpopulations. *Lancet* 574-575.

Bartrop, R.W., Luckhurst, E., Lazarus, L., Kiloh, L.G. & Penny, R. (1977). Depressed lymphocyte function after bereavement. *Lancet 1*:834-836.

Blalock, J.E. & Smith, E.M. (1985b). A complete regulatory loop between the immune and neuroendocrine systems. *Fed. Proc.* 44:108-111.

Butcher, E.C. (1986). The regulation of lymphocyte traffic. *Current Topics in Microbiology and Immunology* 128:85-122.

Claman ,H.N. (1983). Glucocorticoids 1: Antiinflammatory mechanisms. *Hosp. Practice* 123-134.

Cohen, J.J. & Crnic, L.S. (1984). Behavior, stress and lymphocyte recirculation. In: Cooper , E.L. (Ed.) *Stress, Immunity, and Aging*. Marcel Dekker, New York, pp 73-80.

Cohen, J.J. (1987). Immunity and behavior. *Journal of Allergy and Clinical Immunology* 79:2-5.

Crary, B., Borysenko, M., Sutherland, D.C., Kutz, I., Borysenko, J.Z. & Benson, H. (1983a). Decrease in mitogen responsiveness of mononuclear cells from peripheral blood after epinephrine administrations in humans. *J. Immunol.* 130:694-697.

Crary, B., Hauser, S.L., Borysenko, M., Kutz, I., Hoban, C., Weiner, H.L. & Benson, H. (1983b). Epinephrine-induced changes in distribution of lymphocyte subsets in peripheral blood in humans. *J. Immunol.* 131:1178-1181.

Dougherty, T.F. & Frank, J.A. (1985). The quantitative and qualitative responses of blood lymphocytes to stress stimuli. *J. Lab. Clin. Med.* 1953, 42. Reprinted in: Locke, S., Ader, R., Besedovsky, H., Solomon, G., Strom, T. (Eds.) *Foundations of psychoneuroimmunology*. Aldine, New York, pp. 79-86.

Fittschen, B., Schulz, K.-H., Schulz, H., Raedler, A. & Kerekjarto, M.v. (1989). Langfristiger Streß und Herpes-simplex-Antikörper bei gesunden Probanden. In: Speidel, H. & Strauß, B. (Eds.). *Zukunftsaufgaben der psychosomatischen Medizin,* Springer, Berlin, pp. 167-180.

Fittschen, B., Schulz, K.-H., Schulz, H., Raedler, A. & Kerekjarto, M.v. (1990). Changes of immunological parameters in healthy subjects under examination stress. *International Journal of Neuroscience* 51: 3-4.

Fitzgerald, L. (1988). Exercise and the immune system. *Immunol. Today* 9:337-339.

Fleshner, M., Laudenslager, M.L., Simons, L. & Maier, S.F. (1988). Impaired antibody production associated with defeat in rats. *Soc. Neurosci. Abstr.* 14:1283.

Gilman, S.C., Schwartz, J.M., Milner, R.J., Bloom, F.E. & Feldman, J.D. (1982). b-endorphin enhances lymphocyte proliferative responses. *Proc. Natl. Acad. Sci. USA.* 79:4226-4230.

Golub, E.S. (1987). Peers, press, and public: a cautionary note. *Brain, Behavior, and Immunity* 1:195-196.

Guillemin, R., Cohn, M. & Melnechuk, T. (Eds.) (1985). *Neural modulation of immunity.* Raven Press, New York.

Heijnen, C.J. & Ballieux, R.E. (1986). Influence of opioid peptides on the immune system. *Advances* 3:114-121.

Heijnen, C.J., Zijlstra, J., Kavelaars, A., Croiset, G. & Ballieux, R.E. (1987). Modulation of the immune response by POMC-derived peptides. *Brain, Behavior, and Immunity* 1:284-291.

Irwin, M., Vale, W. & Britton, K.T. (1987). Central corticotropin-releasing factor suppresses natural killer cytotoxicity. *Brain Behav. Immunity* 1:81-87.

Irwin, M., Hauger, R.L., Brown, M. & Britton, K.T. (1988). CRF activates autonomic nervous system and reduces natural killer cytotoxicity. *Am. J. Physiol.* 255:R744-R747.

Jankovic, B.D., Markovic, B.M. & Spector, N.H. (Eds.) (1987). Neuroimmune interactions: Proceedings of the Second International Workshop on Neuroimmunomodulation. *Annals of the New York Academy of Sciences, Vol. 496.* New York Academy of Sciences, New York.

Jessop, J.J., Gale, K. & Bayer, B.M. (1987). Enhancement of rat lymphocyte proliferation after prolonged exposure to stress. *Journal of Neuroimmunology* 16:261-271.

Keller, S.E., Weiss, J.M., Schleifer, S.J., Miller, N.E. & Stein, M.(1983). Stress-induced suppression of immunity in adrenalectomized rats. *Science* 221:1301-1304.

Keller, S.E., Schleifer, S.J., Liotta, A.S., Bond, R.N., Farhoody, N. & Stein, M. (1988). Stress-induced alterations of immunity in hypophysectomized rats. *Proc. Natl. Acad. Sci.* USA 85:9297-9301.

Kiecolt-Glaser, J.K., Garner, W., Speicher, C., Penn, G.M., Holliday, B.S. & Glaser, R. (1984). Psychosocial modifiers of immunocompetence in medical students. *Psychosomatic Medicine* 46:7-14.

Kiecolt-Glaser, J.K., Fisher, L., Ogrocki, P., Stout, J.C., Speicher, C.E. & Glaser, R. (1987). Marital quality, marital disruption, and immune function. *Psychosom. Med.* 49:13-34.

Kiecolt-Glaser, J.K., Kennedy, S., Malkoff, S., Fisher, L., Speicher, C.E. & Glaser, R. (1988). Marital discord and immunity in males. *Psychosom. Med.* 50:213-229.

Kiess, W. & Hall, N. (1989). Hormone im Immunsystem. In: Hesch, R.D. (Ed.) *Endokrinologie, Teil A Grundlagen. Innere Medizin der Gegenwart, Bd. 4.* Urban & Schwarzenberg, München.

Kishimoto, T. & Ishizaka, K. (1976). Regulation of the antibody response *in vitro*. X. Bisphasic effect of cyclic AMP on the secondary anti-hapten antibody response to antiimmunoglobulin and enhancing soluble factor. *J. Immunol.* 116:534-541.

Kiss, A., Ferenci, P., Graninger, W., Pamperl, H., Pötzi, R. & Meryn, S. (1983). Endotoxaemia following colonoscopy. *Endoscopy* 15:24-26.

Laudenslager, M.L., Ryan, S.M., Drugan, R.C., Hyson, R.L. & Maier, S.F. (1983). Coping and immunosuppression: Inescapable but not escapable shock suppresses lymphocyte proliferation. *Science* 211:568-570.

Laudenslager, M.L., Fleshner, M., Hofstadter, P., Held, P.E., Simons, L. & Maier, S.F. (1988). Suppression of specific antibody production by inescapable shock: Stability under varying conditions. *Brain Behavior, and Immunity* 2:92-101.

Lenz, H.J., Raedler, A., Greten, G. & Brown, M.R. (1987). CRF initiates biological actions within the brain that are observed in response to stress. *Am. J. Physiol:* 252:R34-R39.

Lenz, H.J. (1987). Extrapituitary effects of corticotropin releasing factor. *Hormone metab. Res. (Suppl.)* 16:17-23.

Levitt, D. & Cooper, M.D. (1987). B-cells. In: Stites, D.P., Stobo, J.D. & Wells, J.V. (Eds.) *Basic and clinical immunology*. Appleton & Lange, Los Altos, pp. 72-81

Locke, S., Ader, R., Besedovsky, H., Solomon, G. & Strom, T. (1985). *Foundations of psychoneuroimmunology*. Aldine, New York.

Maier, S.F. & Laudenslager, M.L. (1988). Inescapable shock, shock controllability, and mitogen stimulated lymphocyte proliferation. *Brain, Behav. Immunity* 2:87-91.

McCain, H.E., Lamster, I.B., Bozzone, J.M. & Grbic, J.T. (1982). b-Endorphin modulates human immune activity via non-opiate receptor mechanisms. *Life Sciences* 31:1619-1624.

Monjan, A.A. & Collector, M.M. (1977). Stress-induced modulation of the immune response. *Science* 196:307-308.

Odio, M., Goliszek, A., Brodish, A. & Ricardo, M.J. (1986). Impairment of immune function after cessation of long-term chronic stress. *Immunology Letters* 13:25-31.

Ovadia, H., Lubetzki-Korn, I. & Abramsky, O. (1987). Characterization of dopamine binding sites on isolated membranes of rat lymphocytes. *Ann. NY Acad. Sci.* 496:211-216.

Raedler, A., Fraenkel, S., Klose, G. & Thiele, H.G. (1985a). Elevated number of peripheral T-cells in inflammatory bowel disease displaying T9 antigen and Fc-alpha-receptors. *Clin. Exp. Immunol.* 60:518-524.

Raelder, A., Fraenkel, S., Klose, G., Seyfarth, K. & Thiele, H.G. (1985b). Involvement of the immune system in the pathogenesis of Crohn's disease: Expression of the T9-antigen on peripheral immunocytes correlates with the severity of the disease. *Gastroenterology* 88:978-983.

Raedler, A., Schulz, K.-H., Bredow, G. & Greten, H. (1985c). Flowcytometrische Bestimmung aktivierter peripherer T-Zellen als Verlaufsparameter beim Morbus Crohn. *Klinische Wochenschrift 63, Suppl. IV*, 123.

Raedler, A., Bredow, G., Kirch, W., Thiele, H.G. & Greten, H. (1986). In vivo activated peripheral T-cells in autoimmune disease. *J. Clin. Lab. Immunol.* 19:181-186.

Raedler, A., Studtman, A., Emskoetter, T., Schulz, K.-H., Greten, H., Fuchs, D. & Wachter, H. (1987). Correlation of urinary neopterin and activated peripheral lymphocytes in inflammatory bowel disease, immunovasculitis and myasthenia gravis. In: Pfleiderer W., Wachter, H. & Blair, J.A. (Eds.) *Biochemical and clinical aspects of pteridines.* De Gruyter, Berlin, pp. 203-212.

Sanders, V.M. & Munson, A.E. (1985). Norepinephrine and the antibody response. *Pharmacol. Rev.* 229-248.

Sapolsky, R., Rivier, C., Yamamoto, G., Plotsky, P. & Vale, W. (1987). Interleukin-1 stimulates the secretion of hypothalamic corticotropin releasing factor. *Science* 238:522-524.

Schleifer, S.J., Keller, S.E., Camerino, M., Thornton, J.C. & Stein, M. (1983). Suppression of lymphocyte stimulation following bereavement. *JAMA* 250:374-377.

Schulz, H., Schulz, K.-H., Fittschen, B., Zeichner, D., Raedler, A., Kerekjarto, M.v. (1989a). Zum Zusammenhang chronischer und akuter Belastung mit immunologischen Veränderungen. In: Laireiter, A., Mackinger, H. (Eds.) *Verhaltensmedizin - Gesundheits-medizin.* Mackinger Verlag, 110-132.

Schulz, K.-H., Lenz, H.J., Messmer, A., Siemen, R. & Raedler, A. (1989b). Charakterisierung blastisch transformierter Immunocyten nach intrathekaler CRF-Injektion bei Ratten mittels monoklonaler Antikörper. In: Speidel, H. & Straub, B. (Eds.) *Zukunfts-aufgaben der psychosomatischen Medizin* . Springer, Berlin 157-166.

Schulz, K.-H. & Schulz, H. Overview of psychoneuroimmunological studies in humans with emphasis on the uses of immunological parameters. In: Jankovic, B.D. (Ed.) *Immuno-Neuro-Endocrine-Network: Recent Research.* Gordon and Breach, New York (in press).

Selye, H. (1976). *Stress in health and disease.* Butterworth, Boston.

Simon, H.B. (1984). The immunology of exercise. A brief review. *JAMA* 252:2735-2738.

Taché, Y., Morley, J.E. & Brown, M.R. (Eds.) (1989). *Neuropeptides and stress*. Springer, New York.

Toennesen, E., Toennesen, J. & Christensen, N.J. (1984). Augmentation of cytotoxicity by natural killer (NK) cells after adrenaline administration in man. *Acta. Pathol. Microbiol. Immunol. Scand.* 92:81-83.

Wysocki, L.J. & Sato, V.L. (1978). "Panning" for lymphocytes: a method for cell selction. *Proc. Natl. Acad. Sci. USA* 75:2844-2848.

Chapter 12

Rapid Resetting of the Baroreflex is Part of Behavioral Changes in Cardiovascular Parameters

Axel Brattström
Michael Sonntag
Edgar Appenrodt
Thomas Seidenbecher
Sos Manutscharow
Arne Brattström
Wolfram Schälicke
Corinna Blumenstein

Institute of Physiology
Medical School Magdeburg, FRG

Institute of Neurobiology and Brain Research
Academy of Science Magdeburg, FRG

Central Institute of Cardiovascular Research
Academy of Science Berlin, FRG

Every change in the internal or external environment challenges somatic as well as psychological responses. Reactions in heart rate and blood pressure are components of a complex and integrated physiological response by which blood supply becomes adapted on demand. When considering blood pressure (BP) both short-term and long-term regulation have to be taken into account, with the former being thought to keep the actual BP within the range which is required for long-term regulation. Consequently, short-term regulation should be subjected to an operational adjustment aimed at setting its operating point at the value required for long-term regulation (Brattström, 1981; Brattström et al., 1985; Brattström, 1988; Conway et al., 1983; Dorward & Korner, 1987; Fritsch et al., 1989; Guyton et al., 1973; Schlör et al., 1984; Walgenbach & Donald, 1983). Short-term regulation of BP mainly refers to baroreflex control. Estimation of the baroreflex under different circumstances has already revealed alterations of this reflex in arterial hypertension, in changed endocrine state or during behavior supporting this suggestion (Dorward & Korner, 1987; Imai et al., 1983; Stephenson, 1984). However, sometimes the reported data were not restricted to real short-term regulation. Moreover, centrally induced BP changes might be mediated by distinguished pathways, and consequently the operational adjustment of the baroreflex might also be distinct. Therefore, the experiments reported here aimed to gain more insight into a possible relationship between centrally induced BP elevation and operational adjustment of the baroreflex. In animals, BP elevation is often induced by intracerebro-ventricular (i.c.v.) administration of either hypertonic saline (HS), angiotensin II (AN II) or the substance P (SP) (Appenrodt et al., 1989; Kawano & Ferrario, 1984; Philippu, 1988; Unger et al., 1988). Whilst i.c.v. administration of HS and AN II activates the central vasopressin system (Ganten et al., 1983ong; Gruber & Eskridge, 1986; Philippu, 1988), SP rather induces an increase in sympathetic drive with a cardiovascular pattern similar to defense reaction (Philippu, 1988; Unger et al., 1988).

In anaesthetized rats (1.3 g urethan/kg) BP, heart period (inter-beat-interval: IBI) and splanchnic nerve activity (SNA considered efferent sympathetic activity) were simultaneously recorded. HS (1 MOL solution) and AN II (20 ng/μl) were i.c.v. infused by means of a pump (0.5 μl/min for 20 min) whilst SP (10 μg/10 μl) was administered as a bolus injection.

BP increased after i.c.v. SP and BS, but remained unchanged with AN II in the dosage used (Fig. 1). IBI became shortened by SP, prolonged by AN II, and by HS it was prolonged at first and then returned to baseline. SNA was strongly increased after i.c.v. SP, was only moderately reduced by AN II, and with HS the initial reduction turned to an increase 15 min after the start of i.c.v. infusion. The distinct reaction patterns of the parameters (BP, IBI, SNA) suggest that the used compounds may recruit different central mechanisms and, therefore, long-term regulation of BP may also use different pathways rather than a common pathway.

In order to describe short-term regulation under the different circumstances the baroreflex control was tested on two occasions, first 10 min before and second 15 min after i.c.v. treat-

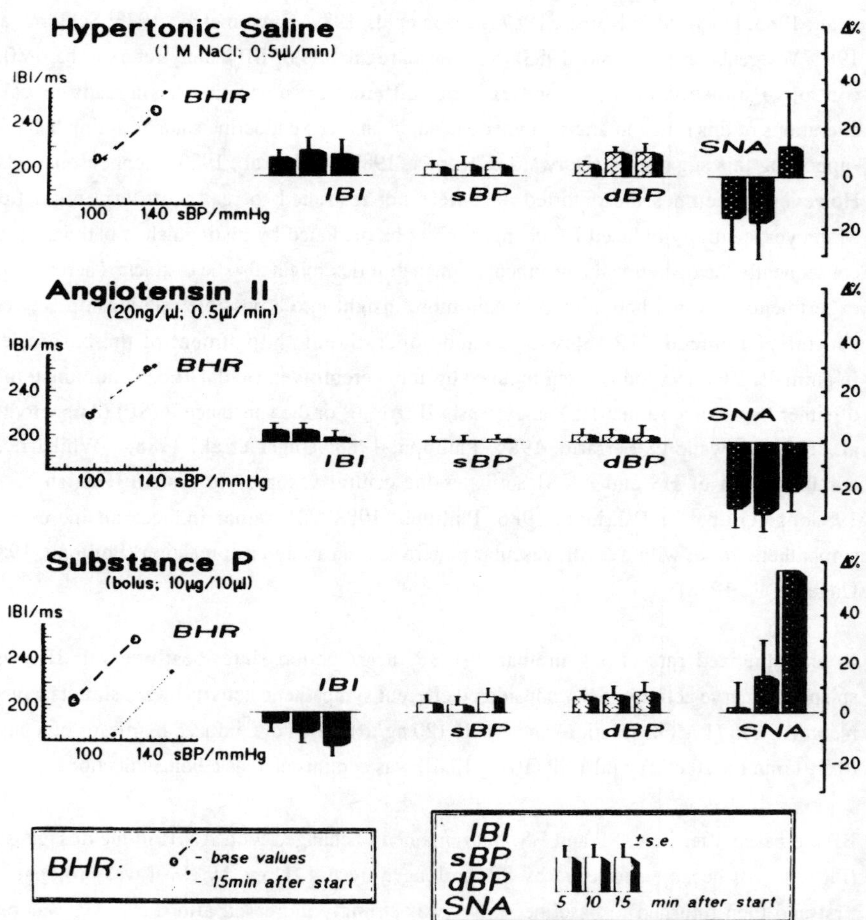

Fig. 1: Cardiovascular responses to i.c.v. administration of HS, AN II and SP. On the left hand side, the BHR are shown 10 min before and 15 min after beginning of i.c.v. treatment, N.B. similarity in gain although IBI and SNA were different at both moments.

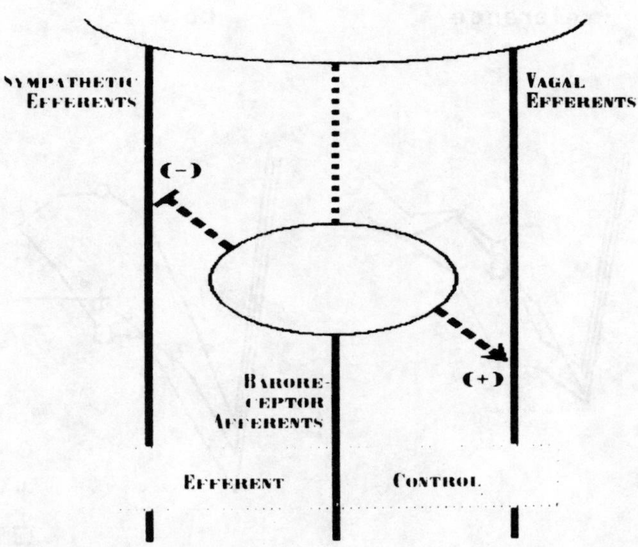

Fig. 2: Schematic drawing of baroreflex actions on brain stem level evoked by an acute BP rise. Incoming baroreceptor afferents inhibit sympathetic efferents as well as exciting parasympathetic (vagal) efferents.

ment. The baroreflex was checked in the following manner: BP was elevated by an intravenous bolus injection of a pressor agent (either 1 - 3 µg phenylephrine or 20 µg methoxa- mine in 10 µl 0.9% NaCl within 10 s) and the reflex prolongation of IBI (so-called baroreceptor-heart-reflex: BHR) as well as the inhibition of SNA estimated (Fig. 2). The gain in the BHR was identical before and after i.c.v. administration of any tested compounds, however, the operating point of the BHR was clearly reset in the case of SP where BP had been elevated (Fig. 1). With regard to the reflex inhibition of SNA a similar figure resulted (Fig. 3), i.e. the normalized reactions before and after i.c.v. treatment were similar although the SNA was different 15 min after i.c.v. treatment (SP ≠; AN II Ø ; HS ≠). In conclusion, under the reported experimental conditions, short-term regulation (reflex prolongation of IBI [parasympathetic component, 24] as well as SNA inhibition [sympathetic component, 241]) behave similarly before and after i.c.v. administration although the reacting parameters (IBI, SNA) have already been changed by long-term regulation.

The afferent traffic from the arterial and cardial baroreceptors terminates in the nucleus tractus solitarius (NTS) of the medulla oblongata. The NTS also receives inputs from other nerves and

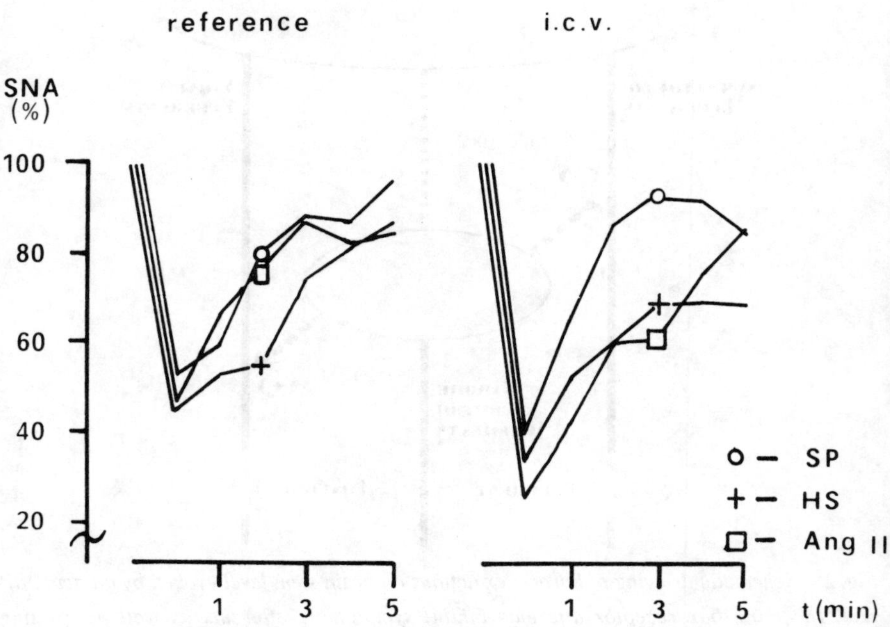

Fig. 3: Baroreflex inhibition of splanchnic nerve activity (SNA) evoked by an acute BP rise within reference period and 15 min after beginning i.c.v. treatment.

from different brain structures, e.g. amygdala and hypothalamus (Kannan & Koizumi, 1988; Nosaka et al., 1989; Veening et al., 1984), making it an important integrating center for the baroreflex control of arterial BP. These morphological findings raise the question of whether or not the NTS might be the site where such an operational adjustment of the baroreflex could take place. Therefore, in another series of experiments in anaesthetized rats either angiotensin III (AN III) or vasopressin (AVP) in the low picogram range were bilaterally microinjected into the NTS (100 pg in 4 µl artificial cerebrospinal fluid). Both of these neuropeptides and also their binding sites have been detected within the NTS. AVP lowered BP and prolonged IBI (5,6), whilst AN III (as AN II does) transiently prolonged IBI only. The BHR, when checked 10 min after microinjection of AVP, was shifted toward lower pressure, i.e. reset without change in sensitivity whilst AN III (as AN II does) reduced the sensitivity of the BHR without resetting it (Fig. 4). These observations indicate that neuropeptides in the low picogram range (considered physiological range) might mediate central adjustment of baroreflex regulation at this site.

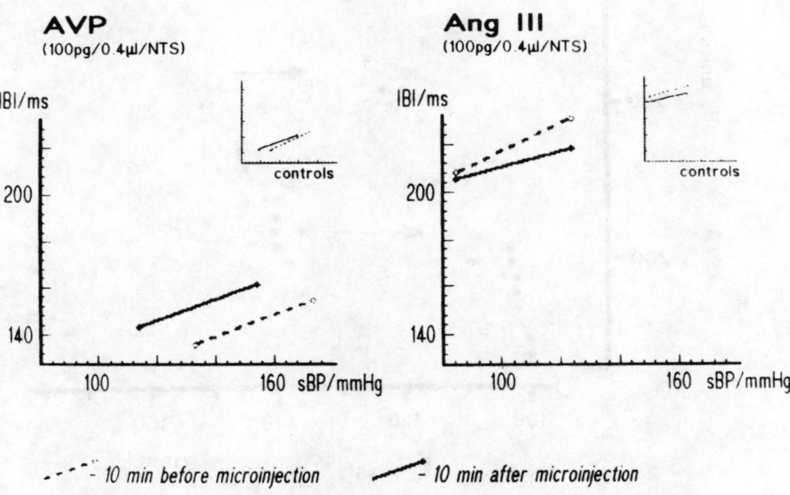

Fig. 4: Baroreceptor-heart-reflex 10 min before and 10 min after bilateral microinjection into the NTS of either AVP or AN III. N.B. AVP shifted the curve whilst AN III reduces sensitivity

The arterial baroreceptors have been suggested to be subject to an efferent control process, whereby their working range becomes adjusted (Brattström, 1981; Brattström et al., 1985; Brattström, 1988; Dorward & Korner, 1987). Therefore, in a third series of experiments in anaesthetized rabbits the aortic baroreceptors were investigated to see whether or not a central induced BP change would be accompanied by such resetting of the baroreceptor working range. For characterization of the aortic baroreceptors the compound potentials of the left aortic nerve (aortic nerve activity; ANA) were plotted against the systolic BP by which they were evoked. The BP in the aortic arch was additionally manipulated by inflation and respective deflation of a small balloon catheter in the abdominal aorta to get a set of BP and ANA data for building up a characteristic function. Two different types of experiment were performed. In a first group of animals the amygdala central nucleus was electrically stimulated (6-8 cps; 2 ms; 0.2-1.5 mA) and the BP was thereby decreased whilst heart rate and respiration remained unaffected (Brattström et al., 1985). The characteristic function of the aortic baroreceptors was shifted toward lower BP, i.e. completely reset without changes in sensitivity 2 min from start of the stimulation period (Fig. 5-A). In a second group of rabbits 30 µg SP were i.c.v. administered to get a central mediated BP rise. The characteristic function of the arterial baro-

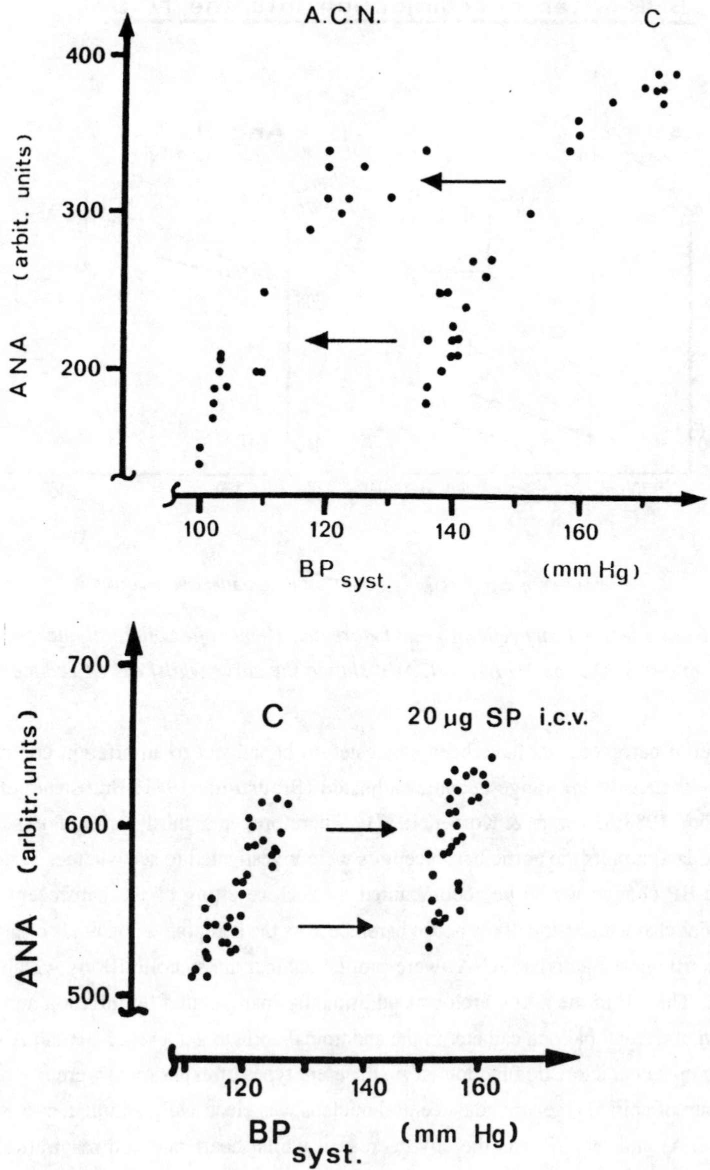

Fig. 5: Aortic nerve activity (ANA) responses to BP increase before (C) and after either lowered arterial BP by electrical stimulation of amygdala central nucleus (ACN) or increased arterial BP by i.c.v. 20 μg SP.

receptors again indicated reset of the baroreceptor working range, however, in this case toward higher BP (Fig. 5-B). In both cases the magnitude of the working range shift corresponded to the change in BP without any loss of sensitivity.

Taken together, BP, IBI and SNA are twofold regulated, i.e. by short-term as well as by long-term regulation. For this reason, changes in these parameters could not be atttributed, at first glance, to one or the other type of regulation, i.e. short-term regulation needs to be checked separately. The presented results clearly indicate that short-term regulation was preserved, although the parameters were also altered by mechanisms of the long-term regulation. Furthermore, this has proven to be true despite the fact that different central pathways were activated. On the other hand, different activation of central pathways may be a useful tool for investigating distinguishable stress-related endocrine and immune responses (Felten et al., 1988; Guyton et al., 1973; Johnson & Torres, 1988; Solomon, 1987).

References

Appenrodt, E., Brattström, A., Moritz, V. & Schälike, W. (1989). Blood pressure and heart rate responses to intracerebroventricular infusion of sodium chloride solution in normotensive and hypertensive rats. *Arch. Int. Pharmacodyn.* 298:68.

Brattström, A. (1981). Modification of carotid baroreceptor function by electriccal stimulation of the ganglioglomerular nerve. *J. Auton. Nerv. Syst.* 4:81.

Brattström, A., Schmidt, D., Oswald, V., Reim, G., Gross, V. & Orlow, G. (1985). Baroreceptor adaptation at different levels of arterial blood pressure. *Rehabilitacia* 30/31:143.

Brattström, A. (1988). Adjustment of the baroreceptor working range. *Activ. Nerv. Sup.* 30:220.

Brattström, A., DeJong, W. & DeWied, D. (1988). Vasopressin microinjections into the nucleus tractus solitarii decreases heart rate and blood pressure in anaesthetized rats. *J. Hypertension 6 (Suppl. 4)*: S521.

Brattström, A., DeJong, W., Burbach, J.P.H. & DeWied, D. (1989). Vasopressin, vasopressin fragments and a C-terminal peptide of the vasopressin precursor share cardiovascular effects when microinjected into the nucleus tractus solitarii. *Psychoneuroendocrinology.* 14(6):461-467.

Conway, J., Boon, N., Jones, J.V. & Sleight, P. (1983). Involvement of the baroreceptor reflexes in the changes in blood pressure with sleep and mental arousal. *Hypertension* 5:746.

Dorward, P.K. & Korner, P.I. (1987). Does the brain "remember" the absolute blood pressure? *NIPS* 2:10.

Felten, S.Y., Felten, D.L., Bellinger, D.L, Carlson, S.L., Ackerman, K.D., Madden, K.S., Olschowka, J.A. & Livnat S. (1988).Nonadrenergic sympathetic innervation of lymphoid organs. *Prog. Allergy* 43:14.

Fritsch, J.M., Rea, R.F. & Eckberg D.L. (1989). Carotid baroreflex resetting during drug induced arterial pressure changes in humans. *Am. J. Physiol.* 256:R549.

Ganton, D., Herman, K., Bayer, C., Unger, T. & Lang, R.E. (1983). Angiotensin synthesis in the brain and increased turnover in hypertensive rats. *Science* 221: 869-871.

Gruber, K.A. & Eskridge, S.L. (1986). Activation of the central vasopressin system: a common pathway for several centrally pressure agents. *Am. J. Physiol.* 251:R476.

Guyton, A.C., Jones, C.E. & Coleman, T.G. (1973). *Circulatory physiology: cardiac output and its regulation.* Saunders Comp., Philadelphia-London-Toronto, 2nd edition.

Hathaway, D.R. & March, K.L. (1989). Molecular cardiology: new avenues for the diagnosis and treatment of cardiovascular diseases. *JACC* 13:265.

Imai, Y., Nolan, P.L. & Johnston, C.I. (1983).Endogenous vasopressin modulates the baroreflex sensitivity in rats. *Clin. Exp. Pharmacol. Physiol.* 10:289.

Johnson, H.M. & Torres, B.A. (1988). Immuneregulatory properties of neuroendocrine peptide hormones. *Prog. Allergy* 43:37.

Kannan, H. & Koizumi, K. (1981). Pathways between the nucleus tractus solitarius and neurosecretory neurons of the supraoptic nucleus: electrophysiological studies. *Brain Res.* 213:17.

Kawano, Y. & Ferrario, C.M. (1984). Neurohormonal characteristics of cardiovascular response due to intraventricular hypertonic NaC1. *Am. J. Physiol.* 247:H422.

Nosaka, S., Nakase, N. & Murata, K. (1989). Somatosensory and hypothalamic inhibitions of baroreflex vagal bradycardia in rats. *Pflügers Arch.* 413:656.

Philippu A. (1988). Regulation of blood pressure by central neurotransmitters and neuropeptides. *Rev. Physiol. Biochem. Pharmacol.* 111:1.

Schlör, K.H., Stumpf, H. & Stock, G. (1984). Baroreceptor reflex during arousal induced by electrical stimulation of the amygdala or by natural stimuli. *J. Auton. Nerv. Syst.* 10:157.

Solomon, G.F. (1987). Psychoneuroimmunology: interactions between central nervous system and immune system. *J. Neurosci. Res.* 18:1.

Stephenson, R.B. (1984). Modification of reflex regulation of blood pressure by behavior. *Ann. Rev. Physiol.* 46:133.

Stornetta, R.L., Guyenet, P.G. & McCarty, R.C. (1987). Autonomic nerval system control of the heart rate during baroreceptor activation in conscious and anaesthetized rats. *J. Auton. Nerv. Syst.* 20:121.

Unger, T., Carolus, S., Demmert, G., Ganten, D., Lang, R.E., Maser-Gluth, C., Steinberg, H. & Veelken, R. (1988). Substance P induces a cordiovascular defense reaction in the rat: pharmacological characterization. *Circ. Res.* 63:812.

Veening, J.G., Swanson, L.W. & Sawchenko, P.E. (1984). Hypothalamic integration: organisation of the paraventricular and supraoptic nuclei. *Brain Res.* 303:337.

Walgenbach ,S.C. & Donald, D.E. (1983).Inhibition by carotid baroreflex of exercise-induced increases in arterial pressure. *Circ. Res.* 52:253.

Part IV

Conditioning Effects

Chapter 13

Restoration of Immune Function by Olfactory Stimulation with Fragrance

Hedeki Shibata
Ryoichi Fujiwara
Mitsunori Iwamato
Harue Matsuoka
Mitchel Mitsuo Yokoyama

Department of Immunology
Kurume University School of Medicine
Kurume, Japan

Introduction

Aggressive behavior can be experimentally induced by removal of the olfactory bulb in animals (Yoshimura et al,. 1974), and this phenomenon suggests that emotional behavior may be regulated by the olfactory bulb. However, the mechanism by which the olfactory system identifies the numerous number of different odors is unclear, although as foreign molecules odors vary widely in their structure and are readily detectable and discriminated. The olfactory epithelium, where the odor receptor neurons are located, could account for odor detection with a dozen separate receptors which overlap to a varying extent in their reactivity towards different odors (Kashiwayanagi & Kurihara, 1984).

We have previously demonstrated that various forms of stress applied to mice influenced humoral and cellular immune responses (Fujiwara et al., 1985; Fujiwara & Orita, 1987; Fujiwara et al., in press). This study is an attempt to determine the influence of odors on the restoration of emotional, behavioral and biological responses which are altered by stress. An aromatic fragrance was applied to mice showing immunological and behavioral changes induced by high pressure stress. The restoration of the altered phenomena was investigated.

Materials and methods

BALB/c male mice, 8-10 weeks old, were used throughout the experiments and were obtained from the Shizuoka Agricultural Cooperative Association for Laboratory Animals, Shizuoka, Japan.

Spleen cell preparation: The spleen was removed aseptically, the cells finely minced in RFMI 1640 media and then passed through a no. 150 wire mesh. The cells obtained were washed three times in phosphate-buffered saline (PBS; pH, 7.4) and then hemolyzed by adding 0.75% tris-ammonium chloride solution (pH, 7.65). The cells were washed three more times and suspended in RPMI 1640 at a concentration of 1 x 10^7 cells/ml.

Plaque-forming cells (PFC) were measured for sheep red blood cells (SRBC) in *in vivo* and *in vitro* tests. In the PFC test *in vivo*, SRBC (2 x 10^8) were injected into the tail vein of the mouse immediately after exposing it to high pressure stress. Five days after the immunization, the spleen was removed and assessed for anti-SRBC with an IgM PFC test according to the method of Cunningham and Azenberg (Cunningham & Szenberg, 1968). In the PFC test *in vitro*, the spleen of the mouse was removed 24 hrs after the stress and the spleen cells were used for further experiments. The spleen cells were isolated and the cell suspension was divided into two groups. The cells in one of the two groups of suspension cells were used as regulator cells and were treated with 25 μg/ml mitomycin C (MMC) at 37°C for 30 min. The MMC-treated cell suspension was mixed with a spleen cell suspension from non-stressed mice and a SRBC suspension. The cell suspension was adjusted to an equal concentration of 5 x 10^6/cell. The cells in the second group of suspension cells were used as effector cells and were mixed with a suspension of SRBC. The mixture was then cultured for 5 days according to the method of Mishell and Dutton (1967) and assayed for PFC. The cell mixture was cultured in RPMI 1640 supplemented with 26 mM HEPES, 300 μg/ml L-glutamine, 100 μg/ml streptomycin, 5 x 10^{-5}M 2-mercaptoethanol and 10% fetal bovine serum (FBS).

A chamber (diameter 125 mm, length 180 mm, volume $2210cm^3$) was used in applying high pressure to the mice. Three mice were put into one chamber and exposed to 2.2 kg/cm^3

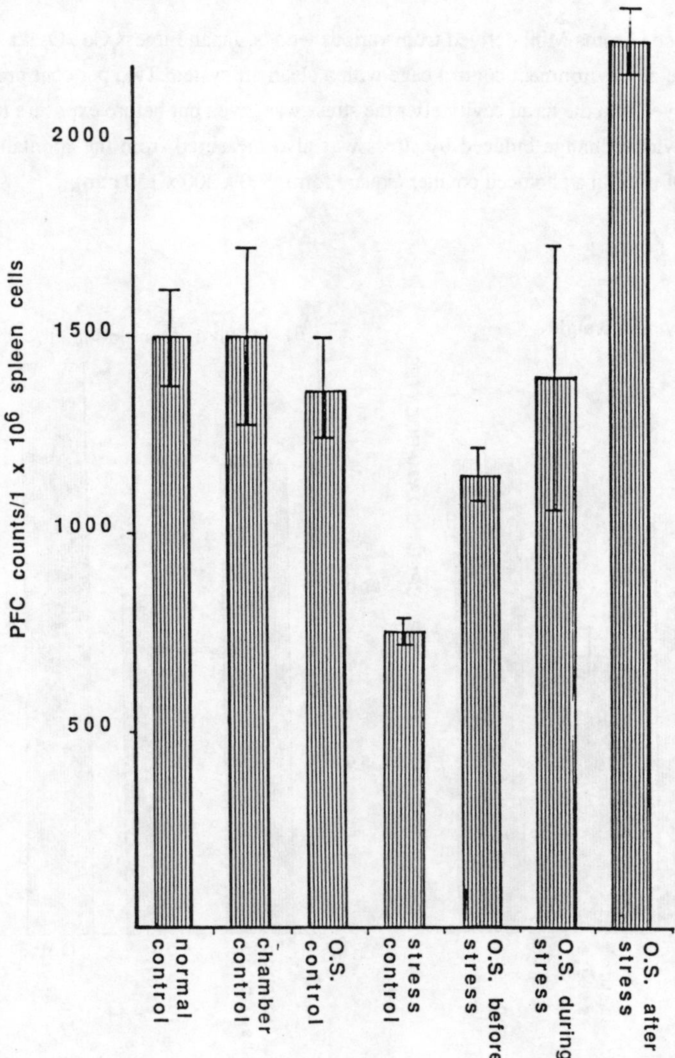

Fig. 1: Effects of fragrance (O.S.) on PFC counts in mice suppressed by high pressure stress on day 5. PFC counts were enhanced by exposing the mice to the fragrance before, during and after the stress.

pressure of compressed air for 60 min, once a day for 2 days. Control mice were placed in this chamber without exposure to pressure.

Aromatic fragrance (Aroma Mini derived from various woods, Japan Fitness Co., Osaka) was applied to mice in an environment control cage with a clean air system.Two per cent procain solution was sprayed into the nasal cavity after the stress was given but before exposure to the fragrance. Behavioral change induced by stress was also measured from the spontaneous running activity of mice in a photocell counter (square form, 300 x 300 x 150 mm).

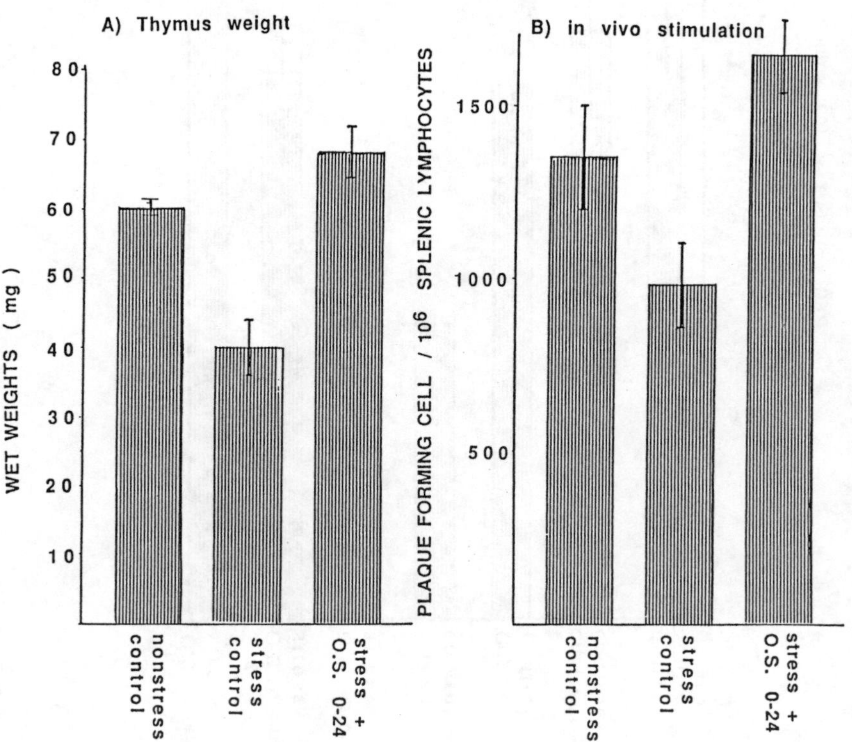

Fig. 2: Effect of fragrance (O.S.) applied for 24 hrs immediately after the stress was given. The thymic involution (a) and the suppression of PFC production (b) induced by high pressure stress was observed on day 5. The thymic involution and ***in vivo*** *PFC production were reconstituted by the exposure to fragrance.*

Results

Mice were injected with SRBC immediately after the exposure to high pressure stress, and a significant reduction of PFC in the spleen cells was observed on day 5 (Fig. 1). However, PFC was restored by exposing the mice to the fragrance before and during stress. In the case of exposure to the fragrance after stress, PFC was markedly enhanced. Mice immunized with SRBC immediately after the stress was given were exposed to the fragrance for 24 hrs, and the *in vivo* PFC test on day 5 was completely restored to the control level (Fig. 2). Thymic involution displayed by the mice after stress recovered with exposure to fragrance.

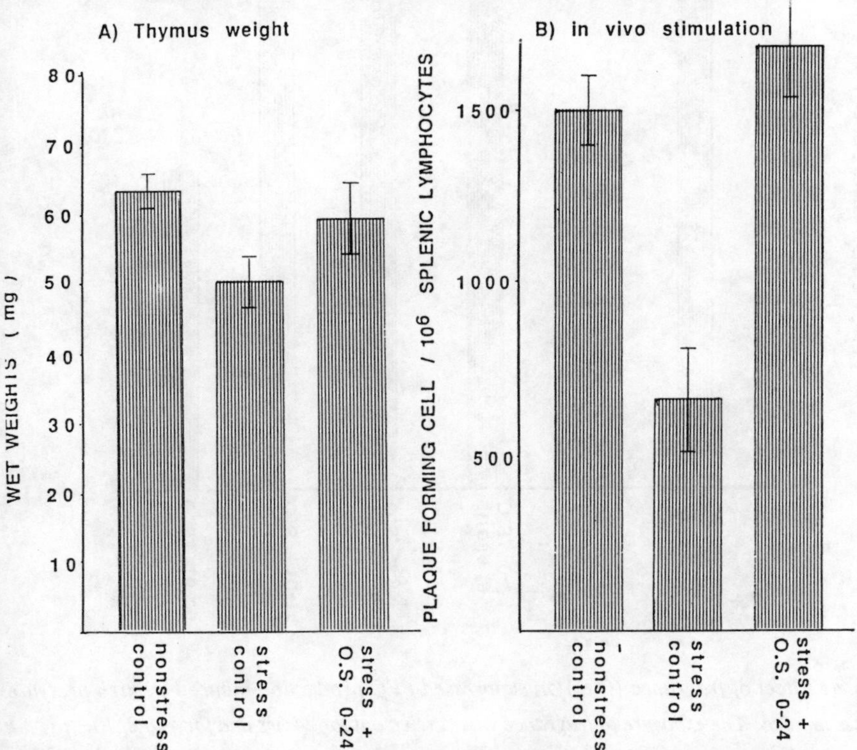

Fig. 3: Effects of fragrance (O.S.) on thymic involution (a) and suppressed PFC production (b) induced by high pressure stress in mice. The thymic involution was observed 24 hrs after the stress and the thymus weight had recovered to some extent through exposure to the fragrance for 24 hrs after the stress. In the ***in vitro*** *PFC test, the PFC count of spleen cells (effector cells) cultured with spleen cells (responder cells) of non-stressed mice for 4 days stress and the count tested on day 5 had recovered through the exposure to fragrance for 24 hrs after the stress.*

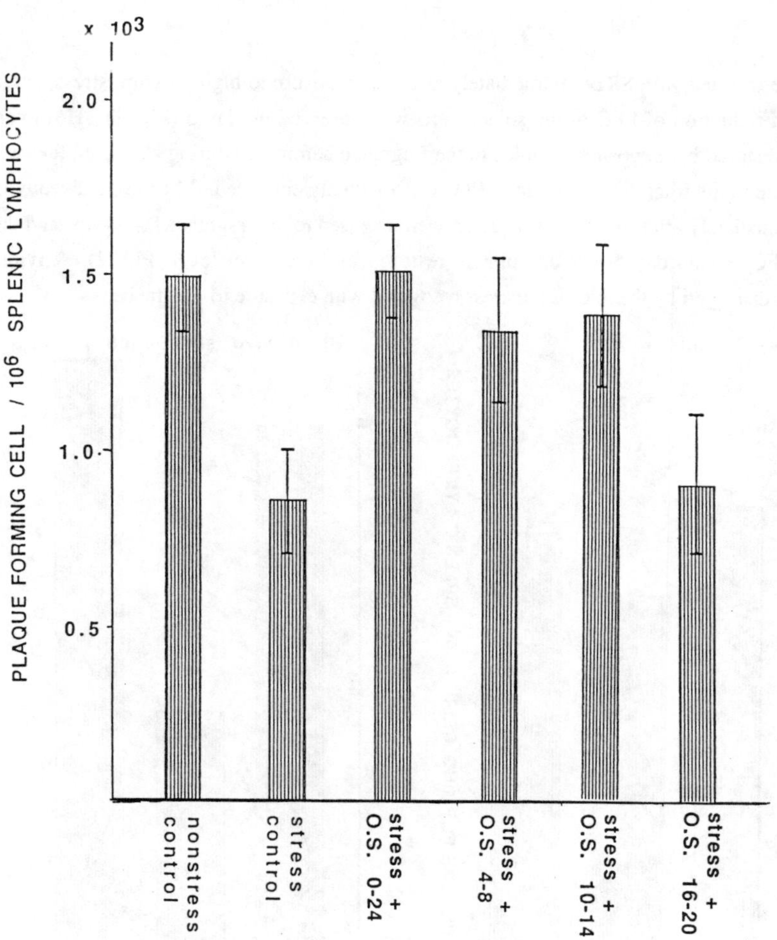

Fig. 4: Effect of fragrance (O.S.) on suppressed PFC production induced by high pressure stress in mice. The exposure to fragrance was carried out for 24 hrs and for 4 to 8, 10 to 14 and 16 to 20 hr periods after stress was given.

The effect of the fragrance on suppressed PFC production induced by high pressure stress was studied *in vitro*, and the spleen cells of mice with suppressor activity for PFC production appeared 24 hrs after the high pressure stress. However, suppressor activity in the spleen cells and thymic involution disappeared after mice were exposed to the fragrance for 24 hrs after the given stress (Fig. 3).

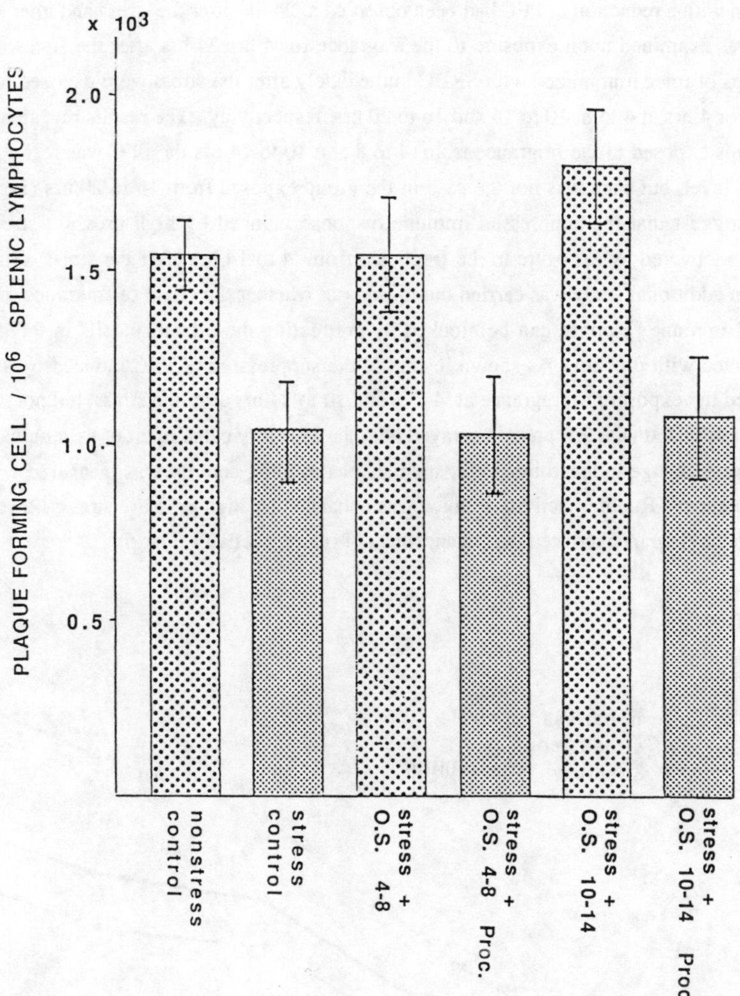

Fig. 5: Effects of procain on suppressed PFC production in mice, restored by exposure to fragrance. The exposure to fragrance for 4 to 8 and 10 to 14 hr periods after the stress did not affect PFC production after procain was administered.

In order to demonstrate the effect of fragrance on immune suppression of reducing PFC induced by high pressure stress, the duration of exposure to the fragrance was experimentally designed. Exposure to the fragrance was carried out at 4 hrs and 24 hrs, respectively, after the high pressure stress. According to a previous experiment (Shibata et al., 1989), immune suppression with a reduction in PFC had been observed at 24 hrs after the stress and, therefore, the PFC was examined upon exposure to the fragrance for 4 hrs 24 hrs after the stress. The three groups of mice immunized with SRBC immediately after the stress were exposed to the fragrance for 4 hrs at 4 to 8, 10 to 14 and 16 to 20 hrs, respectively. The results revealed that in the groups exposed to the fragrance from 4 to 8 and 10 to 14 hrs the PFC was restored to the normal level, but such was not the case in the group exposed from 16 to 20 hrs (Fig. 4). The data suggest that the suppressed immune response induced by high pressure stress is apparently recovered by exposure to the fragrance from 4 to 14 hrs after the stress. Subsequently, an additional study was carried out to find out whether the effect of fragrance on the suppressed immune response can be blocked by pretreating the olfactory cells in the nasal cavity of mice with procain. As shown in Fig. 5, the suppression of PFC induced by stress was blocked by exposure to fragrance at 4 to 8 and 10 to 14 hrs after the stress, but not when mice were pretreated with 2% procain sprayed onto the olfactory cells. In order to demonstrate the behavioral change induced by stress, spontaneous running activity was measured with a photocell counter. Running activity in mice was enhanced by high pressure stress; however, exposure to the fragrance reduced the enhancement of running activity (Fig. 6).

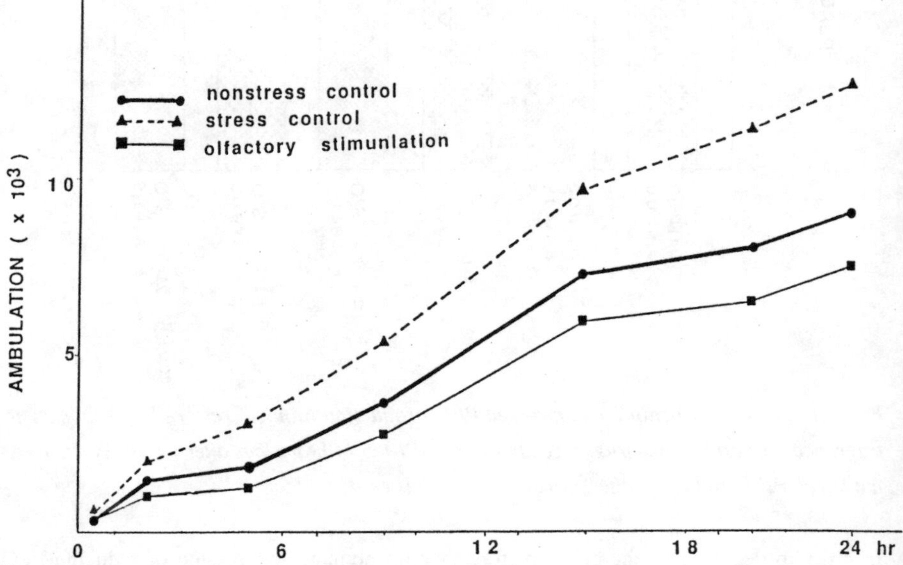

Fig. 6: Effects of fragrance (O.S.) on the enhancement of spontaneous running activity induced by high pressure stress in mice.

Discussion

It could be considered from the results that exposure to an aromatic fragrance blocked the suppression of the immune response induced by stress through the disappearance of suppressor cells and that the behavioral alteration induced by stress was also blocked by the fragrance.

In the past, many ligands have been handed down from aromatherapy experiments using various aromatic fragrances. However, very little information is provided to prove the efficacy of these ligands scientifically. For example, Rovesti and Colombo (Rovesti & Colombo, 1973) reported an improvement in symptoms of anxiety or depression following the sniffing of certain fragrances, e.g. mint, lavender, lemon or jasmin, etc.. They then suggested that the fragrance served as a tranquilizing drug on neuropsychosis. Taneja (Arora et al., 1973) reported that sniffing musk oil inhibited inflammation, although it is well known that inflammatory reaction and the products of inflammation enhance the immune responses (Yoshinaga et al., 1975). In the case of pain stimulation, PFC production was enhanced, but after exposure to fragrance the immune response was normalized (Fujiwara & Orita, 1987). Various stressful events, e.g. inflammation, pain, and neuropsychosis were therefore found to be possibly inhibited by exposure to fragrance. The present results reveal that exposure to fragrance was effective against some forms of physical and emotional stress. We had previously studied (Fujiwara et al., 1985; Fujiwara & Orita, 1987) the influence of pain applied to the neuro-endocrine system on immune responses in mice, and the results clarified that alteration of the immune responses was induced by stimulation of the neuro-endocrine system. The alteration was considered to be due to the activation of regulatory T lymphocytes, helper or suppressor T lymphocytes via mediators from the neuro-endocrine system, e.g. adrenaline or glucocorticoid, etc.. Therefore, responses to stress were divided into two types, one involving thymic involution, the other not. It is known that a thymic involution involving stress suppresses the immune response by activating the suppressor T cells via glucocorticoid (Munster, 1976). It is also known that stress not involving thymic involution enhances the immune response due to activation of helper T cells by adrenaline released from the adrenal gland (Fujiwara et al., 1985; Fujiwara & Orita, 1987). We, therefore, suggest that alteration of the immune response induced by various stresses was due to activation of suppressor or helper T cells via chemical mediators released from the neuro-endocrine system. In this study, stress induced by exposure to high pressure was found to involve thymic involution and to reduce PFC production through the activation of suppressor T cells in mice. As the results reveal, stress involving thymic involution was blocked by exposure to fragrance. We have previously observed (Fujiwara & Orita, 1987) that the enhancement of PFC production induced by stress where no thymic involution is involved, e.g. pain stimulation, is also blocked by fragrance (Shibata et al., 1989). These facts indicate that fragrance could exhibit an anti-stress effect. It is also known that various tranquilizers block the immune suppression induced by stress (Pericic et al., 1987) and that by effecting alteration of the body's biological rhythms they inhibit the emotional disorder induced by stress in the limbic system. This agrees with results demonstrating the non-release of chemical mediators from the neuro-endocrine system (Lister & Nutt, 1986). Similar to the concept mentioned above, it is suggested that the disorder induced by stress was blocked by exposure to the fragrance which modulated the central nervous system. It could also be assumed from these results that nerve fibers (Johnson, 1959) from the olfactory organ were innervated with the limbic system via the olfactory bulb and that olfactory stimulation with aromatic fragrance blocked the activation of the limbic system induced by stress.

References

Arora, R.B., Taneja, V. & Sharma, R.C. (1973). Anti-inflammatory studies on a crystalline steroid isolated from Commiphora mukul. *Indian J. Med. Res.* 60:929-931.

Cunningham ,A.J. & Szenberg, A. (1968). Further improvement in the plaque technique for detecting single antibody forming cells. *Immunology* 14:599.

Fujiwara, R., Tanaka, N. & Orita, K. (1985). Suppressive influence of surgical stress on the graft-versus-host reaction in mice. *Acta. Med. Okayama* 38:439.

Fujiwara, R. & Orita ,K. (1987). The enhancement of the immune response by pain stimulation in mice. *J. Immunol.* 138:3699.

Fujiwara, R., Orita, K., Yokoyama, M.M. (in press) Interactions between the neuro-endocrine and immune system. In: Nistico, G., Masek, K. & Hadden J.W. (Eds.) Pythagora Press, Rome, Italy.

Johnson, T.N. (1959). Studies on the brain of the guinea pig. II The olfactory tracts and fornix. *J. Comp. Neur.* 112:121-139.

Kashiwayanagi, M. & Kurihara, K. (1984). Neuroblastoma cell as a model for olfactory cell; mechanism of depolarization in response to various odorants. *Brain Res:* 293:251.

Kashiwayanagi, M. & Kurihara, K. (1985). Evidence for non-receptor odor discrimination using neuroblastoma cells as a model for olfactory cells. *Brain Res.* 359:97.

Lister, R.G. & Nutt, D.J. (1986). Mice and rats are sensitized to the proconvulsant action of a benzodiazepine-receptor inverse agonist (FG 7142) following a single dose of lorazepam. *Brain Res.* 379:364.

Mishell, R.I. & Dutton, R.W. (1967). Immunization of dissociated spleen cell cultures from normal mice. *J. Exp. Med.* 126:423.

Munster, A.M. (1976). Post-traumatic immunosuppression is due to activation of suppressor T cells. *Lancet* 1, 1329.

Pericic, D., Manev, H., Boranic, M., Poljak-Blazi, M. & Lakic, N. (1987). Effect of diazepam on brain neurotransmitters, plasma corticosterone, and the immune system of stressed rats. *Ann. N.Y. Acad.* 496:450.

Rovesti, P. & Colombo, E. (1973). Aromatherapy and aerosols. *S.P.C. London* 46:475.

Shibata, H., Fujiwara, R., Shichijo, S. & Yokoyama, M.M. (1989). Effect of fragrance on immune suppression induced by the stress in mice. *Clin. Immunol.* 21 (in press).

Yoshimura, H., Gomita, Y. & Ueki, S. (1974). Changes in acetylcholine content in rat brain after bilateral olfactory bulbectomy in relation to mouse-killing behavior. *Pharmacol. Biochem. Behav.* 2:703.

Yoshinaga, M., Nakamura, S. & Hayashi, H. (1975). Interaction between lymphocytes and inflammatory exudate cells. I. Enhancement of thymocyte response to PHA byproducts of polymorphonuclear leukocytes and macrophages. *J. Immunol.* 115: 533.

Chapter 14

Pituitary-Adrenal Influences on Immunoconditioning

Maurice George King
Alan J. Husband
Alexander W. Kusnecov
Diana F. Bull
Richard Brown

Department of Psychology
University of Newcastle, N.S.W., Australia

Pituitary-Adrenal Axis and Immunoconditioning

Our group has been actively engaged in an immunoconditioning program since 1981. An earlier report (King et al., 1987 a) attempted to place in perspective the first five years of our experiments. In this paper, we draw attention to developments in two aspects of that research program which are proving most profitable.

Table 1 summarizes the procedures used in studies of Dexamethasone (DEX) blocking of immunoconditioning (Kusnecov et al., 1988) emanating from our laboratory. The table, though complex, can be more readily understood if it is thought of as one experiment superimposed on another.

Experiment i: The basic taste aversion conditioning design (a Saccharin + Cyclophosphamide Experimental Treatment - Sacc/Cy, 0.15% Sacc in regular drinking water followed 10 mins later by an i.p. injection of 50 mg/kg of CY; a Water + Cyclophosphamide Control Treatment - Wat/Cy, in which the animal's regular drinking water is not flavored with Sacc but the subject

Tab. 1: Experimental procedure for Dexamethasone blockade of immunoconditioning.

Treatment	DEX/PBS Subgroup	Day of Treatment				
		Day 0		Day 2		Day 3
		0400h	0800h	0400h	0800h	0800h
SACC/CY	PBS-PBS	PBS ip	SACC + CY ip	PBS ip	SACC + PBS ip	Assay
WAT/CY		"	Water + CY ip	"	Water + CY ip	"
SACC/PBS		"	SACC + PBS ip	"	SACC + PBS ip	"
SACC/CY	PBS-DEX	PBS ip	SACC + CY ip	DEX ip	SACC + PBS ip	Assay
WAT/CY		"	Water + CY ip	"	Water + PBS ip	"
SACC/PBS		"	SACC + PBS ip	"	SACC + PBS ip	"
SACC/CY	DEX-PBS	DEX ip	SACC + CY ip	PBS ip	SACC + PBS ip	Assay
WAT/CY		"	Water + CY ip	"	Water + PBX ip	"
SACC/PBS		"	SACC + PBS ip	"	SACC + PBS ip	"
SACC/CY	DEX-DEX	DEX ip	SACC + CY ip	DEX ip	SACC + PBS ip	Assay
WAT/CY		"	Water + CY ip	"	Water + PBS ip	"
SACC/PBS		"	SACC + PBS ip	"	SACC + PBS ip	"

does receive the injection of CY; and a Saccharin + Phosphate buffered saline Control Treatment - Sacc/Pbs, in which the animal drinks Sacc flavored water and receives a control injection of Pbs. Conditioning takes place on Day 0 of Table 1; Testing is carried out on Day 2 after which animals are sacrificed for various assays.

Experiment ii: DEX (100 μg/kg i.p. 4 hrs prior) blockade or its Control (Phosphate buffered saline - PBS) is superimposed on the conditioned taste/immunoconditioning in a 2 x 2 design: before Conditioning and before Testing with the CS-alone (DEX-DEX); before Conditioning but not before Testing (DEX-PBS); not prior to Conditioning but before Testing (PBS-DEX) and, finally, no Dexamethasone (PBS-PBS). At the dose of DEX chosen Kusnecov et al. (1989 a) reported approximately 70% reduction of the corticosterone response to ether stress which represents a reduction of massive proportions. The same dose of DEX, however, had no effect on the immune parameters measured.

The individual studies, of which there are several, have been reported elsewhere in detail (Kusnecov et al., 1988). Therefore, it is more appropriate that an appraisal of the overall picture be made; such a summary is attempted in Table 2.

The most general observation is that DEX blockage had no effect whatever on any phase of the taste aversion but it did affect immunoconditioning. This raises the very important question of the linkage between the cognitive/taste conditioning on the one hand and the immunoconditioning on the other, which we have addressed more fully in our recent review of the area (Kusnecov et al., 1989 a). The short empirical answer would seem to be that some UCSs condition better within a Taste Aversion Procedure, others within a strictly Pavlovian Procedure while many UCSs are equally effective in either procedure.

The right hand panel of Table 2 focuses on the immunoconditioning and suggests a failure in acquisition induced by DEX but no effect on retrieval: (i) DEX prior to conditioning results in the failure to establish conditioned immunosuppression, and (ii) DEX does not appear to affect the retrieval of an already acquired CS-immunoCR connection. Although the pattern of results is suggestive of a DEX-induced failure to acquire the immunoconditioned response we conducted further conditioning studies (see below) to test a competing explanation, viz., that the CS-immunoCR connection is established but is masked or abrogated by the DEX pre-treatment.

Tab: 2: Effects of Dexamethasone blockade on conditioned taste aversion and conditioned immunosuppression.

Conditioned Taste Aversion				Conditioned Immunosuppression			
		Pre-Test	Dex			Pre-Test	Dex
		√	x			√	x
Pre-Conditioning DEX	√	Nil	Nil	Pre-Conditioning DEX	√	-ve	-ve
	x	Nil	Nil		x	Nil	Nil

In our report of the DEX study several conditioned immune parameters were included: Immunoglobulin production (IgG, IgM); spleen cell proliferation induced by the mitogens Pokeweed (PWM), Phytohaemagglutinin (PHA) and Concanavalin A (ConA)). The immunity data set generated is difficult to encapsulate and what follows is no alternative to reading the original studies. The taste aversion effects are as simple as the immune effects are complex. The mitogen-induced proliferation of spleen cells is the more persuasive data set. Animals not exposed to DEX provide the bench-mark: the PBS-PBS groups showed strong conditioned immunosuppression which is consistent with other data from this laboratory. More specifically, the proliferation of spleen cells cultured with mitogens (PWM or PHA) was significantly lower in the conditioned animals, i.e., Sacc/Cy vs. Wat/Cy and/or Sacc/Pbs. (The results arising from ConA are not consistent with other data from this laboratory in that this mitogen failed to distinguish the conditioned animals from the controls. Since they do not sway the argument either way we will concentrate here on the PWM and PHA outcomes).

PWM results: Planned comparison of the proliferative responses to PWM in the Sacc/Cy and the Wat/Cy groups using a one-tailed independent t-test revealed that the proliferative response of Sacc/Cy animals was significantly lower than the Wat/Cy group ($p < 0.01$) in animals not receiving DEX treat ment, but was found to differ from the Wat/Cy group in any of the groups receiving DEX whether before or after conditioning. Further analysis of the PWM data using ANOVA revealed a significant main effect of Treatment Group only ($p < 0.001$). This was due to the markedly lower responsiveness of the Cy groups relative to the Sacc/Pbs group in all DEX/PBS pretreatment conditions as assessed by *post hoc* comparisons of group means

(Sacc/Pbs vs. Sacc/Cy: $p < 0.01$ in each condition; Sacc/Pbs vs. Wat/Cy: $p < 0.01$ for DEX-PBS and DEX-DEX conditions.

PHA results: a 2-way ANOVA of the proliferative response to PHA revealed significant differences for the following effects: Treatment Group ($p < 0.001$), DEX-pretreatment ($p < 0.001$) and Group x DEX ($p < 0.001$). For animals not receiving DEX treatment (PBS-PBS) the response of Sacc/Cy animals was significantly lower than that attributable to the residual CY effects displayed by the Wat/Cy group ($p < 0.01$). There were no differences between the Sacc/Cy and Wat/Cy animals for any of the groups receiving DEX. Post hoc analysis of the PHA data revealed that in the PBS-PBS condition the Sacc/Pbs was significantly different from the Sacc/Cy group only ($p < 0.05$). In the DEX-DEX condition both CY groups were significantly different from the Sacc/Pbs group ($p < 0.01$). The main statistical effect of DEX-treatment was due to a significant difference between the PBS-PBS and the DEX-PBS subgroups in the Sacc/Cy treatment ($p < 0.05$) and the PBS-PBS and DEX-DEX subgroups in the Wat/Cy treatment group ($p < 0.01$).

Discussion: The proliferation results revealed that the response of spleen cells from Sacc/Cy animals which did not receive DEX (i.e., PBS-PBS) was significantly lower than that of the critical Wat/Cy controls. Diminished responsiveness to PWM and PHA was observed among Sacc/Cy conditioned animals relative to Wat/Cy animals. (Contrary to expectation ConA did not distinguish between conditioned and control animals).

IgG Results: There were no significant differences between the IgG means.

IgM Results: A 2-way ANOVA revealed significant main effects of Treatment Group ($p < 0.001$) and DEX-pretreatment ($p < 0.01$). Post hoc comparisons revealed that in the PBS-PBS condition, the Sacc/Cy group, but not the Wat/Cy group, was significantly different from the Sacc/Pbs group ($p < 0.01$, one-tailed). Similarly, in the PBS-DEX condition the reduction in the IgM response of spleen cells from the Sacc/Cy group was more pronounced ($p < 0.01$ compared to the Sacc/Pbs) than that of the Wat/Cy animals ($p < 0.05$ compared to the Sacc/Pbs group). For the DEX-DEX condition, however, both Sacc/Cy and Wat/Cy differed significantly from the Sacc/Pbs group ($p < 0.05$), there being no differences between the Cy groups and the Sacc/Pbs group in the DEX-PBS condition. The main effect of DEX-pretreatment revealed by the ANOVA was due to the significantly lower levels of IgM in the DEX-DEX subgroup of Wat/Cy animals ($p < 0.05$), and the lower response of Sacc/Pbs animals pretreated with DEX on the conditioning day ($p < 0.05$). On the IgG assay neither conditioning nor DEX differentiated between the means. By contrast, IgM results were susceptible to conditioning and the conditioned suppression was absent in conditioned groups pretreated with DEX.

Thus, on the one hand Sacc/Cy conditioning of taste and IgG were not affected by DEX blocking at 100 μg/kg before conditioning. By contrast, conditioned suppression of PWM and PHA were prevented by DEX before conditioning.

The pattern of results points to T cells as the target population for Sacc/Cy immunoconditioning since PHA is predominantly a T cell mitogen and PWM is a T cell dependent B cell mitogen (Stobo & Paul, 1973). It is also well recognized that mitogenic stimulation of murine splenocytes is characterized initially by predominantly IgM-secreting B cells. That IgM was the most susceptible immunoglobulin type to conditioning is also consistent even if the pathway is not yet elucidated. Dexamethasone, ACTH and Beta-Endorphin Dexamethazone, a powerful synthetic glucocorticoid, has a spectrum of hypothalamo-pituitary adrenocortical effects. DEX blockade occurs by feedback onto the hypothalamus-pituitary inhibiting corticotropin (ACTH) and beta-endorphin (B-END).

In vitro effects of Pro-opiomelanocortin fragments, particularly the opiods, in relation to immune function are fairly well understood; the same cannot be said for *in vivo* studies. Only recently, we have shown (Kusnecov et al., 1989 b) that these immunopharmacological effects of B-END are opiate dependent and pertain *in vivo*. The *in vivo* confirmation of immuno-pharmacological effects of ACTH and its related fragments has yet to be reported.

In order to pursue the proposition that DEX was producing its conditioned immunoinhibitory effects via inhibition of pituitary ACTH and B-END a follow-up study was carried out which was a variation of the protocol described in Table 1. The experiment included the following groups: the 1st, 2nd and 7th treatment groups from Table 1, i.e., PBS (Sacc/Cy)PBS; PBS (Wat/Cy)PBS and DEX(Sacc/Cy)PBS. Four further groups were added which varied the DEX(Sacc/Cy)PBS group in which either ACTH (10 μg/kg) or B-END (10 μg/kg) was injected s.c. as follows:

(i) treatment followed that of the above-mentioned 7th group DEX (Sacc/Cy)PBS with an injection of ACTH immediately following CY, i.e., DEX (Sacc/Cy ACTH)PBS.

(ii) treatment as for (i) except that B-END was injected immediately after the CY, i.e., DEX(Sacc/Cy B-END)PBS.

(iii) treatment followed that of the 7th group above DEX(Sacc/Cy)PBS but an injection of ACTH replaced the

iv) treatment followed that of the 7th group above DEX (Sacc/Cy)PBS but an injection of B-END replaced the PBS, i.e., DEX(Sacc/Cy)B-END.

All animals in all groups were tested twice for taste aversion, Day 2 as in Table 1 and again on Day 3; all animals were sacrificed on Day 4.

Results and discussion

As observed in the previous study administration of DEX prior to the conditioning, the DEX(Sacc/Cy)PBS treatment, precluded the conditioned immunosuppression in spleen cell proliferation to PHA. Interestingly, this was reversed in the DEX(Sacc/Cy ACTH)PBS group. These were the animals who went through the regular procedure but received an injection of ACTH following conditioning. This did not apply to the DEX(Sacc/Cy)ACTH treatment, which received its ACTH injection in lieu of testing with Sacc.

The fact that the DEX(Sacc/Cy ACTH)PBS treatment reinstated the conditioned immunosuppression rules out failure to acquire as an explanation of the previous set of data. Rather, it points to a masking by DEX although a further possibility remains: failure to convert from short term to permanent memory reversible by ACTH. The IgM effects reported above failed to replicate although trends were strong. As in Table 2 taste aversion was evident in the PBS(Sacc/Cy)PBS group and in all five DEX-treated groups.

Psychological manipulations of fever

Conditionability of febrile reactions: The power of conditioning procedures in manipulation of various immune parameters has been amply demonstrateed in the last 15 years. Prompted by the success of conditioning procedures with other immunoeffectors we began fairly recently experiments to assess the feasibility of conditioning the febrile component. The breakdown of bacterial cells results in peptidoglycan and lipopolysaccharide (LPS) probably producing their potent febrile effects by inducing the production and release from macrophages of the endogenous pyrogen, Interleukin-1 (IL-1). In our preliminary study (Bull et al., 1990) we first established the time course of fever induced by LPS obtained from Escherica coli. At a dose of 100 µg/kg i.p. in rats a significant elevation of rectal temperature (Dose x Time effect : $p < 0.001$) ensued for 11.5 hrs following injection. The maximum elevation was 1.45^{o}C and occurred between 6.5 and 7.5 hrs post-injection.

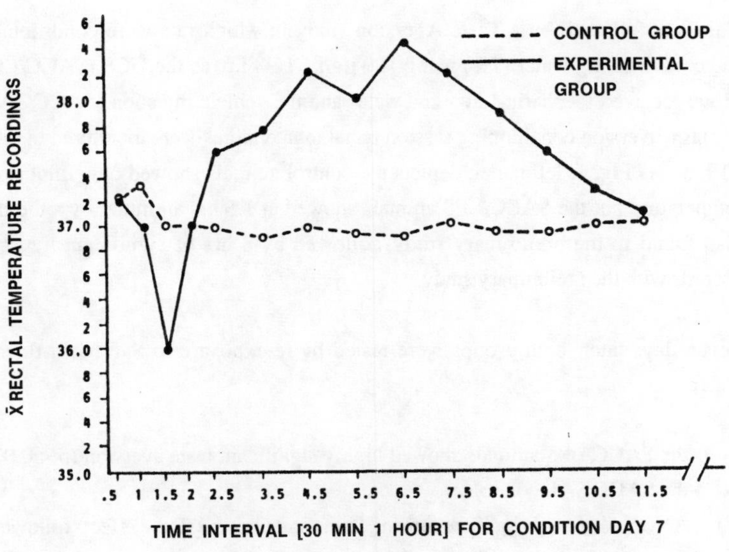

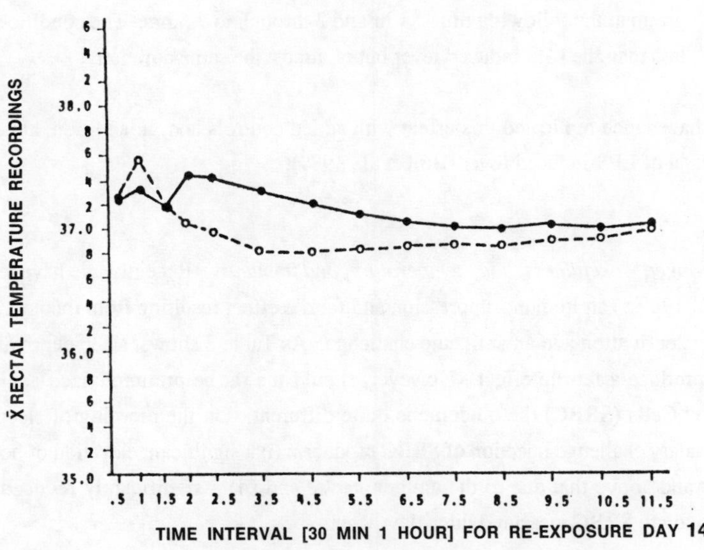

Fig. 1: Rectal temperature conditioning using Lipopolysaccharide as UCS in a taste aversion procedure.

This was followed by a Taste Aversion study in which rats were conditioned to saccharin flavored drinking water (1%) using 100 μg/kg LPS i.p. as the UCS (SACC/LPS). A control group received saccharin-flavoured water and the vehicle injection (SACC/SAL). Following the taste aversion conditioning session rectal temperatures were monitored over the subsequent 11 hrs. As Fig. 1, left panel, depicts the control animals showed only minor perturbations in temperature but the SACC/LPS animals showed at 1.5 hrs an initial hypothermia, which was also found in the preliminary study, followed by 8 hrs of significant hyperthermia which accords with the preliminary study.

Seven days later, both groups were tested by re-exposure to Saccharin-flavoured drinking water.

(i) the SACC/LPS animals showed highly significant taste aversion ($p < 0.0001$) compared to the SACC/SAL controls.

(ii) ANOVA (highly significant main effects and Group x Time effect) followed by *post hoc* analyses revealed that the rectal temperature of the conditioned animals (Fig. 1, right panel) was slightly (but nonetheless significantly) different from the non-conditioned group at the following times: 1 hr and 2 through to 7.5 hrs. The conditioned "fever" was less than the LPS-induced fever but of almost the same duration.

We have since replicated this effect with added controls and, in addition, have conditioned a reversal of LPS-induced fever (Bull et al., 1989).

Prolonged wakefulness, body temperature, and immunity: Recently, we have reported (Brown et al., 1989 a) an immunosuppression and febrile effect resulting from the interaction between sleep deprivation and an antigenic challenge. As Table 3 shows, sleep deprivation alone does not produce a febrile effect. However, should the rat be preimmunized against Sheep Red Blood Cells (SRBC) the outcome is quite different. On the morning of sleep deprivation a secondary challenge injection of SRBC produces: (i) a significant elevation of body temperature over and above that due to the antigen *per se* and (ii) a significantly reduced production of antibody to SRBC measured three days later.

Other data led us to suspect the implication of the endogenous pyrogen, Interleukin-1 beta. Table 3 summarizes the effect of treating the experimental animal with IL-1 (5 or 25 Units) on the morning of sleep deprivation and SRBC challenge. In brief, the febrile effect is countered in the short term and, in the longer term, the deficit in antibody production reverts to normal.

Tab.: 3. Effects of prolonged wakefulness and/or antigenic challenge on antibody production and rectal temperature.

Pre-Treatment	Experimental Treatment	Dependent Variables	Outcome
Handle	Wake8/ Sleep4	Rectal Temp8/4	Normal 8/4
Handle + SRBC	SRBC + Wake8 Sleep4	3 Days: SRBC A'body + Temp8/4	Down Up/Norm4
Handle + SRBC	IL-1(5U) + SRBC + Wake8/ Sleep4	3 Days: SRBC A'body + Temp8/4 +	Normal Normal 8/4
Handle + SRBC	IL-1(25U) + SRBC + Wake8/ Sleep4	3 Days: SRBC A'body + Temp8/4	Normal Normal 8/4

It is not our intention here to go further into these effects. Rather, our aim is to examine neurochemical changes in the hypothalamus accompanying the antibody deficit. At the time when blood was sampled for the SRBC antibody determinations, the hypothalamus was also taken for assay (details of the methods are to be found in (Brown et al., 1989 b).

Table 4 summarizes the hypothalamic levels of indole (Serotonin) and the catecholamines (Norepinephrine and Dopamine) and their metabolites. Of the three transmitters, the serotonergic system was least affected. The precursor Trypotophan, its metabolite and Hydroxy-indoleacetic acid were unaffected by any treatment as was SER itself.

Tyrosine, the precursor for both NE and DA, produced a significant IL-1 effect ($p < 0.05$) and Wakefulness effect ($p < 0.025$). No other NE-related substances were affected including NE itself.

Tab. 4: Mean levels (µg/g tissue, bold print) with Standard Errors (normal print) of neurochemicals in hypothalamus 3 days after prolonged wakefulness.

	TRP	SER	HIAA	TYR	DA	DOPAC	NE	HVA
CON/ SLEEP	4290 222	723 56	378 15	12531 561	503 86	149 44	1592 178	150 19
CON/ WAKE	3990 222	591 56	320 15	12017 788	383 42	89 10	1139 103	130 8
SRBC/ SLEEP	4000 181	667 18	378 11	13342 1219	414 94	114 22	1504 82	113 35
SRBC/ WAKE	4052 135	671 35	378 18	11800 457	292 25	102 14	1432 77	93 7
IL5 SLEEP	4170 178	654 50	373 24	15362 715	351 40	107 9	1331 134	111 7
IL5 WAKE	4226 90	683 23	431 19	12435 532	1041 278	192 39	1258 90	253 33
IL25/ SLEEP	4093 129	720 41	387 23	12133 524	313 67	100 30	1382 114	87 12
IL25/ WAKE	3637 236	656 6	352 13	11215 563	608 104	117 16	1315 48	164 7

Statistically, a strong IL x Sleep effect emerged ($p < 0.006$). A significant increase was evident in the IL-1 (5 units)/Deprived group compared to the IL-1 (5 units)/Sleep group. It is pertinent to note that administration of IL-1 beta to sleeping rats had no effect on DA levels, which suggests that it is the interaction between Wakefulness and IL-1 which produces the DA increase. With respect to the DA metabolite, DOPAC, a significant (IL-1 x Sleep) effect emerged ($p < 0.035$). The IL-1 (5 units)/Wake group had significantly higher levels than the CON/Wake group. With reference to HVA determinations there emerged a highly significant (IL x Sleep) effect ($p < 0.0007$). The IL-1 (5 units/Wake group had 2.5 times more measurable HVA than the IL-IL-1 (5 units)/Sleep group ($p < 0.004$). There was also a significant increase in HVA in the IL-1 (5 units)/Wake group compared to the CON/Sleep ($p < 0.008$) and the SRBC/Wake groups ($p < 0.0001$). The SRBC/Wake group was also significantly lower than the CON/Wake group ($p < 0.004$). This result was also obtained for the IL-1 (25 units)/Wake group which showed significantly higher HVA levels than did the IL25/Sleep group ($p < 0.015$).

The DOPAC:DA ratio showed a highly significant interaction ($p < 0.0025$); the ratio was significantly reduced in the IL-1 (5 units)/Wake compared to the IL-1 (5 units)/Sleep group. The HVA:DA ratio was not affected by any manipulation.

From the above it seems clear that 3 days after the SRBC x Wake treatment, in the hypothalamus, only the dopaminergic system was affected of the three neurotransmitter studies. Almost exclusively, significant changes occurred in relation to the IL-1 and Wake combinations. It is a little surprising that hypothalamic DA was selectively and so profoundly affected. The large increases in DA seen in the IL-1 (5 units)/Wake and to a lesser extent in the IL-1 (25 units)/Wake group suggest that activation of the hypothalamic DA systems can be triggered by an interaction of a behavioral treatment (Prolonged Waking) and an endogenous cytokine.

We regard these findings as a starting point which raise more important questions than they answer. With respect to DA one would wish to know which DA systems were aroused. Another important question is whether the above paradigm is effective with a pathogenic antigen. Recently, we extended the paradigm to study an influenza virus in place of SRBC and found comparable immunological effects (Brown et al., 1989 b). However, the neurochemical profile was swamped by the virus infection *per se*, with all three transmitters being elevated similar to the findings of Dunn et al. (1987), using Newcastle Disease Virus.

References

Bull, D.F., Brown, R., King, M.G. & Husband, A.J. (1990).Modulation of body temperature through taste aversion conditioning. *Physiol. & Behav.* (in press).

Bull, D.F., King, M.G., Pfister, H.P. & Singer, G. (1989). Alpha-melanocyte-stimulating hormone conditioned suppression of a lipopolysacccharide-induced fever. *Peptides* 11:1027-1031.

Brown, R., Price, R.J., King, M.G. & Husband, A.J. (1989 a). Interleukin-1Beta and muramyl dipeptide can prevent decreased antibody responses associated with sleep deprivation. *Brain, Behav. & Immunity* 3: 320-330.

Brown, R., Pang, G., King, M.G. & Husband, A.J. (1989 b).Suppression of immunity to influenza virus infection in the resperatory tract following sleep disturbance. *Regional immunology* 2: 321-325.

Dunn, A.J., Powell, M.L., Moreshead, M.V., Gaskin, J.M. & Hall, N.R. (1987). Effects of the Newcastle Disease virus administration to mice on the metabolism of cerebral biogenic amines, plasmacorticosterone, and lymphocyte proliferation. *Brain, Behav. & Immunity* 1:216-230.

King, M.G., Husband, A.J. & Kusnecov, A.W. (1987). Behavioral conditioning of the immune sytem: from laboratory to clinical application. In: Sheppard, J.L. (Ed.). *Advances in behavioural medicine*. Cumberland, Sydney 4:15.

Kusnecov, A.W., Husband, A.J. & King, M.G. (1988). Behavioral conditioned suppression of mitogen-induced proliferation and immunoglobulin production: Effect of time span between conditioning and re-exposure to the conditioning stimulus. *Brain, Behav. & Immunity* 2:198-211.

Kusnecov, A.W, King, M.G.& Husband, A.J. (1989 a). Immunomodulation via behavioral conditioning. *Biol. Psychol.* 28:25-29.

Kusnecov, A.W., Husband, A.J., King, M.G. & Smith, R. (1989 b).Modulation of mitogen-induced cell profileration and the antibody-forming cell response by Beta-endorphin in vivo. *Peptides* 10:473.

Stobo, J.D. & Paul, W.E. (1973). Functional hetreogenity of murine lymphoid cells. III Differential responsiveness of T cells to phytohemagglutinin and cocanavalin A as a probe for T cell subsets. *J. Immunol.* 110:362.

Chapter 15

Treatment Nausea and Vomiting in Cancer Patients: A Conditioned Reflex?

Gerassimos A. Rigatos

1st Department of Medical Oncology
Athens, Greece

Anticancer chemotherapy is a method of treating malignant tumors which has been in use for almost fifty years. By this therapeutic method a number of cures or complete remissions of the disease with prolonged survival have been achieved for several types of neoplasm. In other cases, too, although the results are not so favourable concerning survival, chemotherapy may be of value in ameliorating various symptoms, e.g. diminution in size of an intrathoracic tumor mass ameliorates dyspnoea, or diminution of a hepatic metastasis diminishes distension of the hepatic capsule and reduces pain.

Certain disadvantages restrict the use of cytostatic drugs, namely, the need for close medical attention, frequent hospitalization, frequent laboratory tests, the cost, and mainly several side effects.

Vomiting and nausea are among the most frequent side effects and the main toxicity in more than a half of cases. Most problematic vomiting is caused by cisplatinum, dacarbazine, dactinomycin, nitrogen mustard, cyclophosphamide, etc. (Gralla et al., 1987). Doctors treating cancer patients are well aware how serious the problem of vomiting can be and how difficult it is to control vomiting with common antiemetics. It is known that the action of cytostatics begins 1 to 2 hrs after administration and lasts from 2 to 24 hrs. In some cases, the emetic effect of chemotherapy may persist for days (Smyth, 1988). Delayed emesis adversely affects the patient's quality of life, can lead to further complications, such as anorexia or inadequate caloric intake, and may affect the physical as well as the psychological condition of the cancer patient.

Data gathered at the University of Rochester Cancer Center and reported recently by Morrow & Dobkin (1988) showed that 60% of 950 consecutive patients under chemotherapy experienced nausea without vomiting, while 40% experienced both nausea and vomiting following the treatment. About one third of the patients in the above-mentioned paper (32%) reported more than severe or severe nausea, while an equal percentage reported moderate nausea, although they had been given the usual antiemetic drugs.

The above data support the common perception of oncologists that nausea and vomiting, despite antiemetic drug intervention, are the more common side effects of cancer treatment.

Pretreatment nausea and vomiting, also called anticipatory (ANV), is a problem which has occupied the interest of oncologists for a decade. It was in 1979 when Scogna & Smalley (1979) gave a clear description of ANV in 41 patients. The following year Nesse et al. (1980) studied the phenomenon in 18 patients with malignant lymphoma. Since then, ANV has been studied in a number of papers.

In this paper we shall provide some observations made among Greek cancer patients, which contribute to the understanding of the phenomenon and support its conditioned nature. These data could also contribute to some conclusions and proposals for the prevention and relief of ANV.

Material and Methods

Our material consisted of 1,020 patients, all with histologically proven types of malignancy. Of the above number, 540 were inpatients and 480 outpatients. In the first group the majority suffered from lung cancer, various types of bone or soft tissue sarcoma and metastatic breast cancer. The majority of the outpatients were suffering from breast cancer. All patients were submitted to various established schedules of combination chemotherapy with 2 to 5 drugs. All of them were given some antiemetic treatment at the same time as chemotherapy. For outpatients or inpatients with minor and less toxic schedules the classic drug metoclopramide was injected intravenously at a dose of 20 mg. For patients receiving more toxic treatment a combination of antiemetic drugs was administered. The combination consisted of methylprednisolone, usually 40 mg every 8 hrs, diazepan, 5 mg every 8 hrs, and chloropromazine, 12.5 mg every 8 hrs. In some cases, metoclopramide was also given in patients prone to rapid nausea and vomiting or for extremely emetogenic schedules.

Results

1. ANV occurred in 316 patients (31%); in 71 of them (7% of the total) the vomiting could be characterized as severe.

2. A direct correlation between highly emetogenic drugs and ANV was documented. ANV was more frequent among patients treated with combinations of dacarbazine, cisplatin and nitrogen mustard.

3. The number of cycles of chemotherapy correlated positively with ANV. Patients undergoing chemotherapy for more than 9 consecutive cycles were twice as likely to experience ANV as patients under therapy for less than six cycles.

4. The same likelihood applied for patients with previous experience of chemotherapy, even if some years earlier.

5. Patients receiving inadequate antiemetic treatment during the few initial cycles of chemotherapy experienced ANV more often.

6. Development of the ANV phenomenon does not seem to be correlated with sex, age and education.

The description of some characteristic cases also supports the conclusion that the nature of this phenomenon is a conditioned response.

Case 1. An 18-year-old male patient, the only child from a family of low socioeconomic background with first grade education, who is suffering from Hodgkin's disease, stage IV. He was treated with the MOPP regimen. After the administration of therapy the young patient vomited, usually 15 to 20 times during the whole day of chemotherapy. After the third course he started vomiting some hours before the phlebocentesis for chemotherapy. After the sixth course, intravenous pyleography was ordered for clinical restaging. Just as the phlebocentesis was complete and before any administration of the radiopaque solution the patient began vomiting and the examination was cancelled.

Case 2. A 48-year-old male patient, a farmer, with splachnic metastases of a bladder carcinoma. The patient had been treated with chemotherapy in the past. When the new chemotherapy schedule began he experienced very severe nausea and vomiting. In the subsequent cycles of chemotherapy the patient had intolerable ANV one or two days before and decided to stop the treatment. It is worthwhile to note that the patient vomited strongly before any communication by telephone with his doctor.

Case 3. A 52-year-old female patient with breast cancer who had been treated with adjuvant chemotherapy in the past. Upon each admission to hospital for reevaluation or other reasons than chemotherapy she vomited when chemotherapy was administered to other patients in the same room.

Case 4. A female patient with special courage towards her disease. She had had a bilateral mastectomy for cancer of the breast, surgical excision of skin metastases and total replacement of the head of the femur for pathologic fractures. Later on she received chemotherapy treatment at home for disseminated disease. She discussed all aspects of her disease freely. After the third cycle of chemotherapy she started to vomit in anticipation of the treatment, Moreover, she vomited whenever she smelt alcohol, because alcohol had been used to disinfect the skin before chemotherapy.

Case 5. A woman with ovarian cancer who was under chemotherapy with a cisplatin combination. The patient used to have only one or two cups of milk before the treatment. At the fourth cycle of chemotherapy and then for a long time after stopping the treatment she experienced nausea at the sight of milk and in special instances even at the thought of it.

Discussion

Some comments could be made concerning our material. The percentage of patients with ANV is of a medium frequency, rates given by various authors ranging widely from 18% (Nicholas, 1982) to 63% (Cella et al., 1984). When, in 1979, Scogna and Smalley (1979) described their patients with ANV they estimated the percentage to be 37% of the total of 41 patients. In the following year Nesse et al. (1980) studied the phenomenon in 18 patients with malignant lymphoma; 8 of them had symptoms of nausea and vomiting before the administration of therapy. The authors supposed this response to be a conditioned one. In the same year Schultz (Schultz, 1990) reported his material with 31% of patients experiencing ANV and explained it as a classical Pavlovian conditioning.

Tab. 1: ANV reported by the 5 larger series of patients.

Authors	No of patients	AN %	AV %	ANV %
Morrow and Dobkin (3)	1250	-	-	25
Morrow (17)	406	24	9	-
Morrow (10)	225	-	-	21
Cohen (9)	149	42	27	-
Love et al. (15)	126	38	-	38

Tab. 2: The highest percentages of ANV reported in literature.

Authors	No of patients	AN %	AV %	ANV %
Cella et al. (7)	60	63	-	-
Weddington (12)	17	53	12	-
Nesse et al. (5)	18	44	-	-
Cohen (9)	149	42	27	-
Nicholas (6)	50	42	-	-
Love et al. (15)	126	38	-	38
Scogna and Smalley (4)	41	-	-	37

Since then, at least 20 papers have described the phenomenon and reported rates of patients who experienced ANV (Scogna & Smalley, 1979; Nesse et al., 1980; Schultz, 1980; Cohen, 1982; Morrow, 1982; Nerenz et al., 1982; Nicholas, 1982; Weddington, 1982; Wilcox et al., 1982; Fetting et al., 1983; Love et al., 1983; Redd et al., 1983; Cella et al., 1984; Morrow, 1984; Van Komen & Redd, 1984; Andrykowski et al., 1985; Dobkin et al., 1985; Dolgan et al., 1988; Morrow & Dobkin, 1988; Smyth, 1988). In Table 1 we summarize the results for the five larger series of patients. The highest percentages of ANV reported in literature are shown in Table 2. The correlation between the emetogenic potential of the drugs and ANV found in our material was also documented by Dolgan et al. (1988), Morrow (1982), and Wilcox et al. (1982).

The longer period of treatment, expressed also by the number of cycles of chemotherapy, was found to correlate positively with ANV. This was also reported by Nesse et al.(1980) who found that patients with ANV were treated for a mean of 9.3 months instead of the 4.2 months of treatment for patients without ANV. This association is supported by data from some other studies. Wilcox et al. (1982) found that patients given more than 9 cycles of chemotherapy had ANV to a percentage of almost 80%. Love et al. (1983) found that patients at the sixth cycle of therapy showed double the percentage of ANV than patients given only two cycles of treatment. The correlation between previous experience of chemotherapy and ANV found in this study has not been demonstrated in other papers as far as we know.

Inadequate antiemetic treatment causes severe post-chemotherapy nausea and vomiting, which in turn cause anxiety. According to Houts et al. (1984) pretreatment anxiety facilitates the conditioning of ANV.

Sex, age and educational status of our material were not correlated with ANV. With regard to sexual status, there is only one study (Fetting et al., 1983) correlating feminine gender with ANV symptomatology. An age younger than 50 has been found in some studies to be correlated with ANV experience (Cohen, 1982; Morrow, 1982; Van Komen & Redd, 1984; Ingle et al., 1984). In similar studies, educational level as well as socioeconomic and marital status were not correlated with ANV.

Various views have been published concerning the etiology of ANV. The physiologic view presupposes brain or gastrointestinal metastases (Chang, 1981). But brain, as well as GI metastases, are of much lower incidence than ANV. Moreover, it has been proven (Morrow & Dobkin, 1988) with randomized clinical studies that there is no such an association between these two parameters.

The psychological aspects, reviewed recently (Morrow & Dobkin, 1988), propose a) a psychodynamic origin, which supposes an underlying psychological readjustment (Chang, 1981); b) a deficiency in the coping mechanisms (Altmaier et al., 1982); c) an involvement of anxiety, initially after the treatment and then anticipatory to treatment (Houts et al., 1984); d) concerning conditioning etiology two models have been discussed. One of them, the operant model, suggests that behaviour develops and continues because it is reinforced. According to the classical model an unconditioned response, post-chemotherapy nausea and vomiting, follows an unconditioned stimulus, the treatment. After a number of repeated cycles of therapy various impressions will become conditioned stimuli, giving a conditioned response (Burish & Carey, 1984). At least one experimental work supports the classical model. In 1978 Bernstein

(1978) in his study with leukaemic children showed that disgust towards a certain kind of ice cream could result if the ice cream was given alongside chemotherapy.

Among our patients we have observed the following conditions acting as conditioned stimuli:

Persons, such as doctors or nurses;
Places, like surgeries, polyclinics or hospital rooms;
Actions, such as phlebocentesis and administration of intravenous infusions;
Smells, like white or blue alcohol, the special smell of chambers and so on;
Tastes, such as special kinds of cream, ice cream, milk, etc.;
Noises, like voices of staff, the rolling of the nursing trolley, even pieces of music, usually broadcast over the special hospital radio system;
Other conditions, such as communication by telephone with the doctor or nurse, admission to hospital, chemotherapy administered to other patients.

Apart from the above-mentioned data the conditioned nature of ANV is supported by the reports of some typical cases (Rigatos, 1985) as well as by a paper examining methods of systematic desensitization for the prevention or reduction of chemotherapy-caused side effects (Dobkin & Morrow, 1988). What we would like to propose for the prevention or reduction of ANV could be summarized as follows:

1. Although treatment of ANV is important, prevention is probably more successful (Gralla, 1988) ANV results mainly from poor antiemetic control during the first few courses of chemotherapy. Thus, a complete antiemetic control during that period is of great value.The strong antiemetic treatment is of more value if chemotherapy is highly emetogenic. Drugs reducing anxiety, such as diazepam or lorazepam, must be included.Chloropromazine (or another phenothiazine) must be used in an antiemetic combination not only because it blocks the chemotherapy receptor trigger zone but also because of its central suppressive action. Corticosteroids must be included also because of their proven antiemetic effect, although the site and mechanisms of action are not established (Freedman, 1986). High dose metoclopramide should be avoided because it is only moderately effective while being severely toxic.

2.The new antiemetic GR 38032 F (Ondansetron) which is a 5-HT_3 antagonist appears to be a promising antiemetic and may reduce not only post-chemotherapy nausea and vomiting but also the ANV (Smyth, 1988).

3. Avoidance of the formation of conditioned reflexes must be our second significant interest. Among these one could also mention both the avoidance of preparation of drugs in front of the patient and of special or characteristic smells, noises, etc..

4. Various methods of systematic desensitization (Dobkin & Morrow, 1988), progressive muscle relaxation, or various psychologic methods of treatment, if possible to apply, should be encouraged and must be of some value, although not yet totally accepted.

References

Altmaier, E.M., Ross, W.E. & Moore, K. (1982). A pilot investigation of the psychologic functioning of patients with anticipatory vomiting. *Cancer* 49:201.

Andrykowski, M.A., Redd, W.H. & Hatfield, A.K. (1985). Development of anticipatory nausea: A prospective analysis. *J. Consult. Clin. Psych.* 53:447.

Bernstein, I.L. (1978). Learned taste aversions in children receiving chemotherapy. *Science* 200:1302.

Burish, T.G. & Carey, M.P. (1984). Conditioned responses to cancer chemotherapy: Etiology and treatment. In: Fox, G.H. & Newberry, B.H. (Eds.) *Impact of psychoendocrine systems in cancer immunity*. Hogrefe, Toronto.

Cella, D.F., Pratt, A. & Holland, J.C. (1984). Long-term conditioned nausea and anxiety persisting in cured Hodgkin´s patients after chemotherapy (Abstract). *Proc. Am. Soc. Clin. Oncol.* 3:73.

Chang, J.C. (1981). Nausea and vomiting in cancer patients. An expression of psychological mechanisms? *Psychosomatics* 22:707.

Cohen, R.E. (1982). *Distress associated with antineoplastic chemotherapy: Prediction, assessment and treatment*. Doctoral Dissertation, State University of New York, Albany.

Dobkin, P.L. & Morrow, G.R. (1988). Prevention of chemotherapy induced nausea and vomiting. In: Lobo A. & Tres A. (Eds.) *Psicosomatica y cancer*. Ministerio de Sanidad, Madrid, p. 197.

Dobkin, P., Zeichner, A. & Dickson-Parnell, B. (1985).Concomitants of anticipatory nausea-emesis in cancer chemotherapy. *Psychol. Rep.* 56:671.

Dolgan, M.J., Katz, E.E., McGinty, K. & Seigel,S.E. (1988). Anticipatory nausea and vomiting in pediatric cancer patients. *Pediatrics* (in press, quoted by 3).

Fernandez-Argüelles, P., Guerrero, J., Dugue, A., Borrego, A. & Marquez, J. (1988). Nauseas y vomitos anticipatorios en patientes cancerosos sometidos a tratamiento de quimioterapia. In: Lobo A. & Tres A. (Eds.). *Psicosomatica y cancer*. Ministerio de Sanidad, Madrid, p. 387.

Fetting, J.H., Wilcox, P.M., Iwata, B.A., Criswell, E.L., Boamajian, L.S. & Sheider, V.R. (1983). Anticipatory nausea and vomiting in ambulatory medical oncology population. *Cancer Treatm. Rep*. 67:1093.

Freedman, R.S. (1986). *The control of chemotherapy induced nausea and emesis*. Upjohn.

Gralla, R.J. (1988). Approaches to management of nausea and vomiting in the clinical setting. *Clinician* 6 (3):26.

Gralla, R.J., Tyson, L.B., Kris, M.G. & Clark, R.A. (1987). The management of chemotherapy-induced nausea and vomiting. *Med. Clin. North Am.* 71: 289.

Houts, P., Morrow, G.R., Lipton, A., Harvery, H.A. & Simmonds, M.A. (1984). *The role of pre-treatment anxiety in anticipatory nausea among cancer patients receiving chemotherapy*. Unpublished manuscript, University of Pittsford (quoted by 3).

Ingle, R.J., Burish, T.G. & Wallston, K.A. (1984). Conditionability of cancer chemotherapy patients. *Oncol. Nurs. For*. 11:97.

Love, R.R., Nerenz, D.R. & Leventhal, H. (1983). Anticipatory nausea and vomiting in ambulatory medical oncology population. *Proc. Amer. Soc. Clin. Oncol.* 1:183.

Morrow, G.R. (1982). Prevalence and correlates of anticipatory nausea and vomiting in chemotherapy patients. *J. Natl. Cancer Inst.* 68:585.

Morrow, G.R. (1984). *Effects of the cognitive hierarchy in the systematic desensitization treatment of anticipatory nausea in cancer patients: A component with relaxation only, counseling and no treatment.* Unpublished manuscript, University of Rochester (quoted by 3).

Morrow, G.R. & Dobkin, P.L. (1988). Biobehavioral aspects of the cancer traetment side effects. In: Lobo A. & Tres A. (Eds.) *Psicosomatica y cancer (6th International Symp. of EUPSYCA Proceedings)* Ministerio de Sanidad, Madrid,.p. 33.

Nerenz, D.R., Leventhal, H., Love, R.R., Coons, H. & Ringler, K. (1982). *Anxiety and taste of drugs during injections as predictors of anticipatory nausea in cancer chemotherapy.* Unpublished manuscript, University of Wisconsin, Madison (quoted by 3).

Nesse, R.M., Carli, T., Curtis, G.G. & Kleinman, P.D. (1980). Pretreatment nausea in cancer chemotherpy: A conditioned response? *Psychosom. Med.* 42:33.

Nicholas, D.R. (1982). Prevalence of anticipatory nausea and emesis in cancer chemotherapy patients. *J. Behav. Med.* 5:461.

Redd, W.H., Rosenberger, P.H. & Hendler, C.S. (1983). Controlling chemotherapy side effects. *Am. J. Clin. Hyp.* 25:161.

Rigatos, G.A. (1985). *Introduction to psychosocial oncology*, Athens (in Greek).

Schultz, L.S. (1980). Classical (Pavlovian) conditioning of nausea and vomiting in cancer chemotherapy (Abstract). *Proc. Am. Soc. Clin. Oncol.* 21:244.

Scogna, D.M. & Smalley, R.V. (1979). Chemotherapy induced nausea and vomiting. *Amer. J. Nurs.* 79:1562.

Smyth, J. (1988). The problem of emesis induced by cancer chemotherapy. *Clinician* 6 (3):2.

Van Komen, R.W. & Redd, W.H. (1984). *Personality and treatment variables associated with anticipatory nausea and vomiting inpatients receiving cancer chemotherapie.* Unpublished manuscript, University of Illinois, Campaign 1984 (quoted by 3).

Weddington, W.W. (1982). Psychogenic nausea and vomiting associated with termination of chemotherapy. Psychother. *Psychosom*. 37:129.

Wilcox, P.M., Fetting, J.H., Netteschein, K.M. & Abeloff, M.D. (1982). Anticipatory vomiting in women receiving cyclophosphamide, methotrexate and 5-FU (CMV) adjuvant chemotherapy for breast carcinoma. *Cancer Treatm. Rep*. 66:1601.

Part V

Stress, Immunity, Cancer, AIDS, and other Pathological Conditions

Chapter 16

Psychological Factors Influencing the Course of Infectious Disease, e.g. Acute Viral Hepatitis

Burdhard F. Klapp
Brigitte Leyendecker
Ursula Bartholomew
Bettina Jesberg
Jörn W. Scheer

Rudolf Virchow University Hospital
Free University of Berlin, F.R.G.

As indicated by the title of this book, psychoneuroimmunology means the investigation of interactions among various systems within an individual, such as the brain, nervous system, immune system, endocrine system and psychological system, as well as interactions between social subsystems, as expressed by behaviour.

Changes within these systems, for which single variables may be indicators, are studied for possible dependence on

- genetic factors
- environmental/interpersonal stressors
- and intrapersonal factors acquired during life (e.g. depression).

Table 1 shows which groups of individuals are generally studied.

Tab. 1: Types of groups studied.

healthy animals	(e.g. Laudenslager et al. 1983, Coe et al. 1987)
sick animals	(e.g. Ader 1982, Ghanta et al. 1985)
healthy humans	(e.g. Kiecolt-Glaser et al. 1986, Kennedy et al. 1988)
sick humans	(e.g. Schleifer et al. 1985, Darko et al. 1988)

The most rarely investigated individuals are *sick humans*. The reason for this is that such studies are subject to various complicating factors:

1. From a methodological point of view, one has to take into account that some of these systems show pathological change and that little is known about mechanisms of reaction under such pathological conditions. Therefore, different starting conditions have to be expected.
2. From an ethical standpoint, experimental designs using psychosocial stressors are extremely limited because the course of disease may be negatively influenced.
3. The history of medical science has produced an understanding of illness as being mainly a biological event. Therefore, this concept dominates medical research, and young researchers are not encouraged to develop integrated approaches.

Despite these discouraging difficulties, however, we are convinced that clinical psychoneuroimmunological studies are now necessary. Following the postulate that psychotherapeutic interventions will have a positive effect on the course of a given disease, they would allow empirical testing of psychoneuroimmunological hypotheses.

These studies should focus on diseases in which immunological pathomechanisms are presently considered to play an important role, such as:

infectious diseases;
cancer;
autoimmune diseases
and allergies.

All four cases have in common that the immune system is malfunctional: an infection is preceded by incompetent defence against microorganisms; in the case of several forms of neoplasia, pathologically transformed cells are not destroyed; autoimmune diseases result from the breakdown of self-tolerance, and in the case of allergies, immunologic reactivity is enhanced.

Our research centres on the psychological and social dimensions of infectious disease, consequently, this paper concentrates on infection.

Some early reports on infectious diseases may today be viewed as precursory "psychoneuroimmunological" studies. Three examples for prospective studies of this kind are:

Calden et al. (1960), who found that the patients with tuberculosis who showed a tendency to depression, hypochondria and social withdrawal recovered more slowly than those with less features of this kind.

Imboden et al. (1961) examined 600 subjects prior to the winter period using various psychological questionnaires. They found that among the subjects who subsequently caught influenza, the ones who tended to be more depressed recovered more slowly.

Kasl et al. (1979) examined US-army cadets with regard to acquisition of mononucleosis. The seroconverters with subsequent illness differed from those without mononucleosis. The former were highly motivated, had over-achieving fathers and poor academic performance.

Table 2 lists the immunologic and psychosocial variables which were related to each other in the three studies named.

These early studies represent mainly clinical-empirical research, in which interrelations between biological, psychological and social variables were examined on the basis of certain hypotheses.

Unfortunately, we have no knowledge of more recent multidimensional clinical studies on patients with infectious disease which correlate immunologic, psychological and social variables. Presently, efforts are being made to establish psychoneuroimmunological approaches towards patients with AIDS, e.g. the long survivors study planned by Solomon et al. (1986).

Tab. 2: Early prospective psychoneuroimmunological studies.

Author	Disease	Immunologic parameter	Psychological and social variables
Calden et al. (1960)	tuberculosis	length of recovery	- depression - hypochondria - social withdrawal
Imboden et al. (1961)	influenza	length of recovery	- tendency towards depression
Kasl et al. (1979)	mononucleosis	illness	- high motivation - poor academic performance - over-achieving fathers

Our study: Hepatitis as a model for psychoneuroimmunological research

We will now present in more detail the complex, multimodal project on psychological and social features of acute viral hepatitis that we conducted in 1983/1984.

There are three reasons why hepatitis is an appropriate object for clinical psychoneuroimmunological studies:

1. Due to the absence of therapeutic regimens, it is possible to observe the original host-parasite interaction.

2. Patients are generally hospitalized for several weeks, have few bodily complaints and are highly responsive.

3. The course of disease varies extremely, hepatitis B and Non-A, non-B hepatitis lead to chronic disease in 5-10% of cases.

Some pathomechanisms involved in hepatitis A and B have been explained recently. It is known, for example, that the liver cells are not destroyed by the virus itself, but by cellular immunological host reactions against the altered cell membrane. Nothing is known about the mechanisms involved in Non-A, non-B hepatitis (Meyer zum Büschenfelde, 1987).

Interestingly, several studies dating back to the time before hepatitis had been identified as an infectious disease report distinctive psychological features of patients with jaundice. For example, it was a common belief that jaundice could develop immediately or shortly after sudden, overwhelming sorrow. This illness was called "icterus ex emotione" (Frerichs, 1858).

The Second World War led to the recognition of hepatitis as a contagious disease. Since then, some authors have paid special attention to the observed depression of patients with hepatitis. This has been attributed to several different causes, including neurotropic features of the virus (Leibowitz & Gorman 1952) or toxic-metabolic (Gidaly et al., 1964), psychoreactive (Kipshagen, 1975) and endogenous factors (Zeichen, 1986). Additionally, Paar et al. (1987) found no evidence for the contrasting hypothesis that hepatitis may be a substitute for depression.

Hypotheses: Own observations led to the hypothesis that, besides biological determinants like the type of virus or the immunologic status of the host, psychosocial factors such as depression

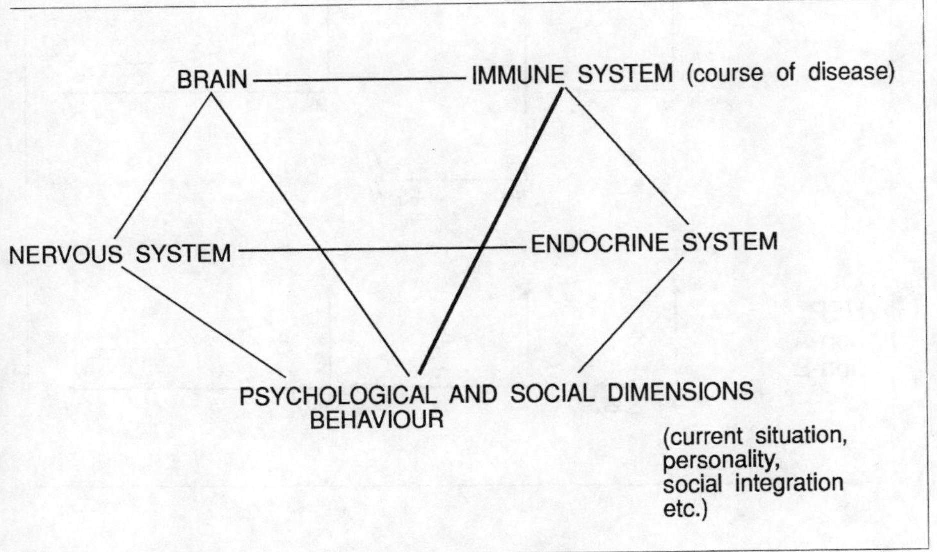

Fig. 1: Interacting systems

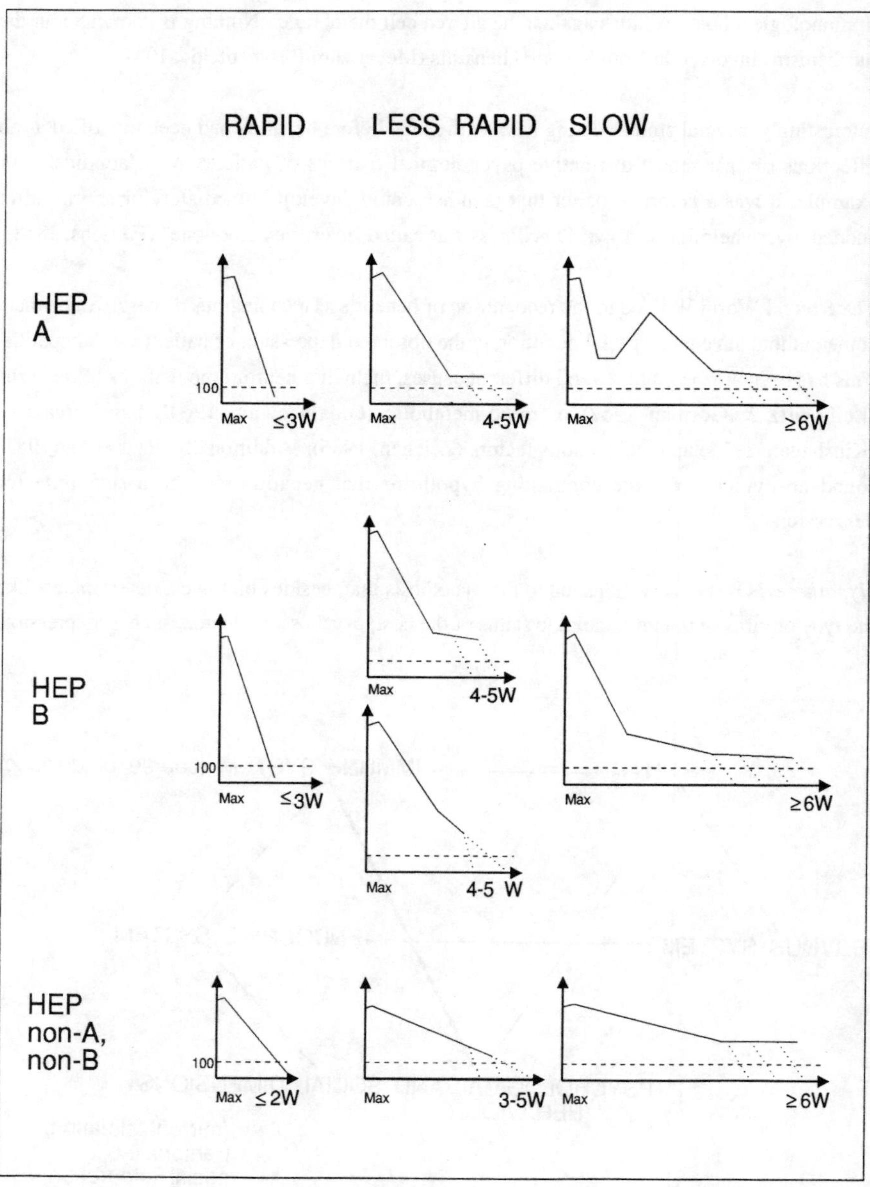

Fig. 2: Differences in the course of disease (ALT)

distress and familial patterns of behaviour could also influence the clinical picture and the course of disease. It was expected that patients with subsequent slow recovery would provoke a clinical impression shortly after admission to hospital and that deleterious behaviour, social stressors and intrapersonal or interpersonal conflict might be involved in their illness.

The study presented is concerned with the interaction between the immunological process and psychological and social dimensions (Fig. 1).

Methods: Subjects were 22 male and 28 female patients, 8 with hepatitis A, 24 with hepatitis B and 18 with Non-A, non-B hepatitis. Average age was 33 years. The individual immunological process was assessed indirectly with the course of the serum transaminase ALT. Subjects were divided into groups representing rapid, less rapid and slow recovery (Fig. 2).

The course of ALT stands for the host's capability to eliminate the virus from the body within a certain period of time, thus terminating liver inflammation. This measure itself is derived from complex relationships between the subsystems of the immune system (humoral and cellular, macrophages, etc.) and the liver cell systems.

We had access to several routinely assessed components of the immune system, from which the following six were chosen for statistical analysis: gamma globulin, immunoglobulins (IgM, IgG, IgA) and autoantibodies (ANA, AMA, SMA), as well as lymphocytes and monocytes.

Tab. 3: Relationships between immunologic function and course of disease.

Finding	Course	Significance
Normal lymphocyte counts / transient lymphocytopenia	rapid recovery	$p \leq 0.05$
Absolute lymphocytopenia of variable duration	slow recovery	
High monocyte counts	slow recovery	$p \leq 0.10$
low monocyte counts	rapid recovery	
Non-A, non-B hepatitis/ high monocyte counts	slow recovery	$p \leq 0.05$
Non-A, non-B hepatitis/ low monocyte counts	rapid recovery	
Hepatitis A/ antinuclear antibodies	slow recovery	

Correlations found between single variables confirmed relationships between the course of ALT and components of the immune system (Table 3).

It was found that the subsequent course of disease was associated with lymphocyte and monocyte counts, the latter correlation being strongest for Non-A, non-B hepatitis. Further, in the case of hepatitis A, slow recovery seemed to correlate with the presence of autoantibodies.

The degree of liver damage during the acute phase did not correlate with the subsequent course of disease.

We attempted to assess subsystems and variables within the *psychological and social dimensions* in a broad set of questionnaires as well as in bedside interviews. The following somatic, psychological and social systems and variables, respectively, were assessed (Table 4):

Tab. 4: Multimodal concept of the hepatitis project.

Processual evaluation of liver damage
Components of the immune system

Prodromi and current bodily complaints
Current mood
Personal experience of hospitalisation

Biographical history
Social situation
Personality
Personal constructs
Life events

Attributes of illness
Coping with illness
Hopes and expectations regarding recovery

Interviewer ratings of communicative behaviour and psychiatric findings
Clinical appraisal
Alexithymic behaviour

Results: In a first step, hypotheses specific to hepatitis were tested by evaluating single questionnaires and somatic variables. Results, thus derived, were used to determine possible relevant biopsychosocial characteristics for this group of patients (Table 5).

Tab. 5: Major characteristics of hepatitis patients.

Dimension	Major characteristics	Methods/remarks
Bodily complaints	2 scales - specific liver complaints - unspecific general complaints	Gießen questionnaire for bodily complaints (GBB), Gießener Beschwerdebogen Brähler and Scheer 1983)
Current mood	6 mood dimensions - anxious depressed - aggressive-tense - weary - concentrated-concerned - vital - untroubled	Multidimensional mood questionnaire (MSF, Mehrdimensionaler Stimmungsfragebogen Hecheltjen and Mertesdorf 1973)
self-concept	- hepatitis patients more depressed than general population 4 personality types - "socially sufficient" - "socially insufficient" - "undercontrolled-hypomanic" - "compulsive-depressed"	Gießen-Test (Beckmann, Brähler and Richter 1983)
	3 groups - high self-esteem - medium self-esteem - low self-esteem 4 self-identity groups - "self satisfied" - "splendid isolated" - "normal" - "isolated"	Role-repertory grid (Kelly 1955) high self-esteem — hypomanic in Gießen-Test low self-esteem — depressed in Gießen-Test

For example, two independent patterns of bodily complaints were found:, specific liver complaints and a complex of non-specific general complaints. The specific liver complaints correlated with the degree of liver damage.

Six major mood dimensions were identified and, according to specific variables derived from the personality questionnaire and the role-repertory grid, it was possible to distinguish between hypomanic, "normal" and depressed patients.

Another interesting result was that the role-repertory grid presented certain patterns of self-perception so far lacking description in the relevant literature, such as "self-satisfaction", "splendid isolation" and "isolation".

Likewise, our first approach towards possible correlations between psychosocial factors and the subsequent course of hepatitis was one-dimensional.

However, as can be seen in Table 6, no relationships were found, apart from the fact that at discharge the patients with rapid recovery felt more weary, less vital and less "concentrated-concerned".

Comprehensive evaluation, however, meaning the connection of various data derived from different dimensions, did not reveal differences between the three recovery groups.

Those patients with a subsequent rapid course reacted to the liver damage initially and predominantly (compared to the other two groups) with liver-specific complaints, which were accompanied by weariness. It is mainly in this group that specific organ damage was associated with an untroubled mood (Fig. 3).

In the case of patients with a subsequent less rapid course of the disease, a connection between liver-specific complaints and organ damage could not be observed. Here, the bodily symptoms were correlated to a greater extent with weariness and low vitality than in the other groups. During the acute phase, the general complaints were associated with "aggressive-tenseness" (Fig. 4).

Tab. 6: Relationships between course of disease and various biopsychosocial dimensions during the acute phase and at discharge.

Dimension	Variable	Acute phase	Discharge
disease variable	liver damage	ns	ns
bodily complaints	liver complaints	ns	ns
	general complaints	ns	ns
mood	anxious-depressed	ns	ns
	aggressive-tense	ns	ns
	weary	ns	(R>IR>S) **
	concentrated- concerned	ns	LR>S>R **
	vital	ns	LR>S>R **
	untroubled	ns	ns
depression	basic mood	ns	-
	self-esteem	ns	-
self-concept	personality types	ns	-
	personality profiles	ns	-
	various other self-concept dimensions	ns	-
interviewer concept of patient	basic mood	ns	-
	personality profiles	ns	-

R = rapid recovery, LR = less rapid recovery, S = slow recovery.

Likewise, in the case of patients with subsequent slow recovery, a relationship between measurable organ damage and characteristic liver complaints was absent. However, liver damage and also jaundice correlated with a "concentrated-concerned" mood. Analogous to the patients with rapid and less rapid recovery, complaints were associated with "weariness". Additionally, however, both the liver-specific and the diffuse non-specific complaints were connected with "anxious-depressiveness" and "aggressive-tenseness" (Fig. 5).

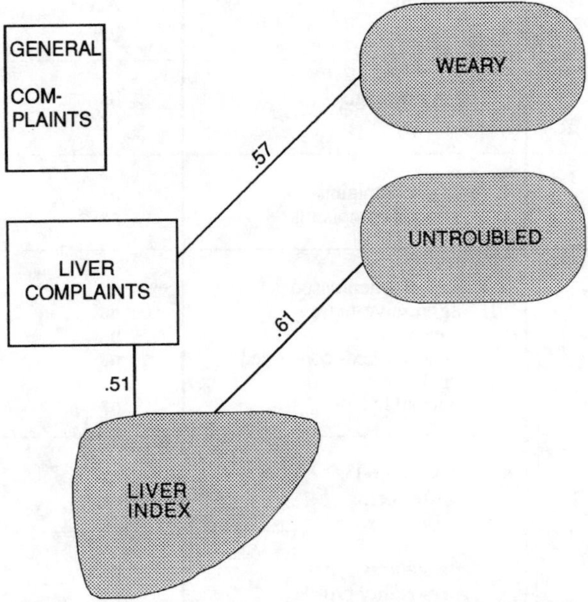

Fig. 3: Significant correlations between bodily complaints, mood, and liver damage for the group with rapid recovery.

Unfortunately, due to limited space, it is not possible to present an interesting case study within which all accessible individual data have been connected and which underlines the fact that a multifactorial event requires a multifactorial approach.

Conclusions and future research

These results confirm our notion that the course of an infectious disease is a complex issue and that, therefore, one-dimensional investigations must naturally fall short. One must abandon the idea that single variables may be used as predictors for the subsequent course of viral hepatitis or, presumably, any other infectious disease.

ACUTE PHASE: LESS RAPID RECOVERY GROUP

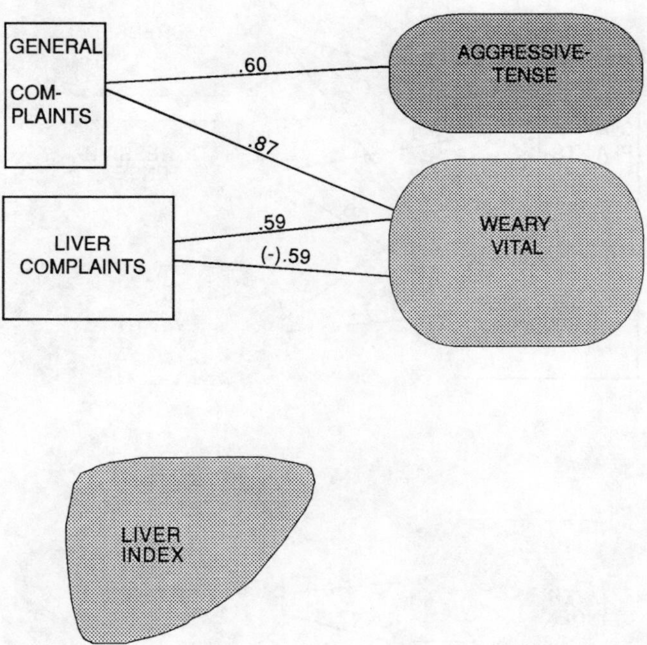

Fig. 4: Significant correlations between bodily complaints, mood, and liver damage for the group with less apid recovery.

In the case of the hepatitis patients, only the combination of various variables allowed a tentative discrimination between three recovery groups.

Bearing in mind our postulate that psychotherapeutic intervention has a positive effect on single components and sub-systems of the immune system or the immune system as a whole, those hepatitis patients who presented that special pattern of mood dimensions and complaints on admission and subsequently showed slow recovery could now be identified as a target group for such an intervention. A body schema-oriented method of therapy, which provides relaxation and relief during the acute phase of the illness, would be most promising in this case.

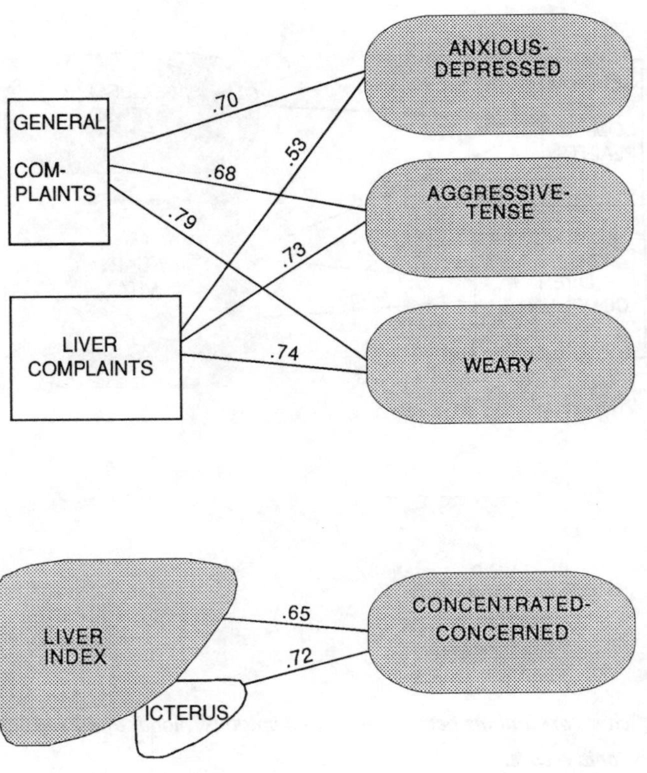

Fig. 5: Significant correlations between bodily complaints, mood, and liver damage for the group with slow recovery.

Currently, we are preparing a broad, controlled, multimodal clinical study in which, as demonstrated in Fig. 6, complex structures within the psychological and social dimensions will be evaluated in combination with the immune system and other systems of the body. Furthermore, the influence of psychotherapeutic interventions will be tested. Goals will be to promote relief from detectable psychosocial stressors and, working at the level of the body schema, to help develop adequate coping and conflict resolving strategies (Fig. 6).

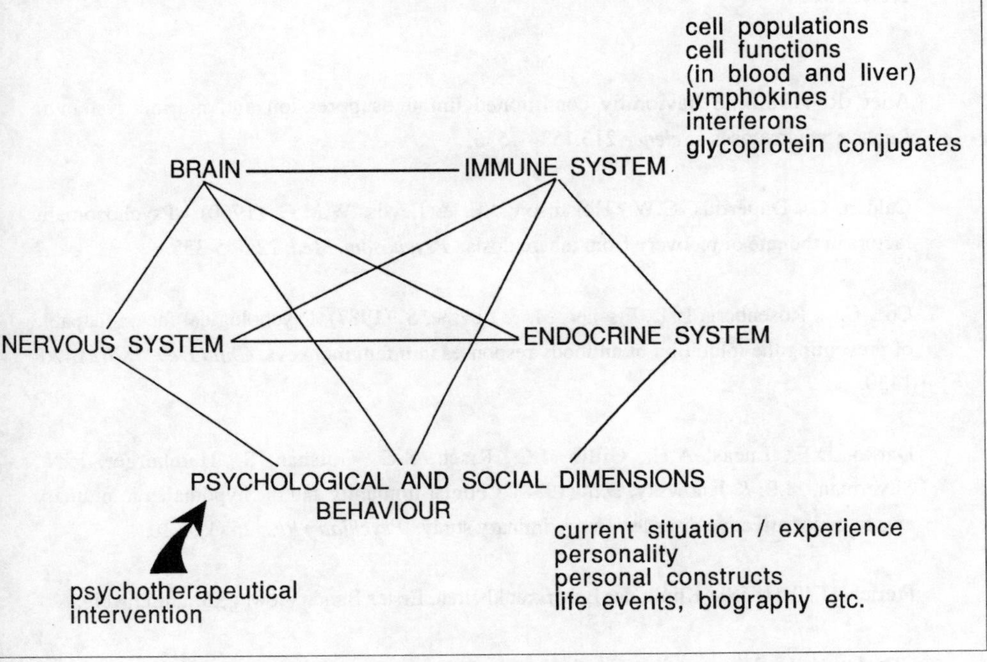

Fig. 6: Interactions to be investigated in a future study.

Thanks to tight cooperation with the Berlin University Institutes for Clinical Chemistry and Immunology, first preliminary studies, e.g. on glycoprotein conjugates in saliva and verbal and preverbal psychotherapy are in process.

References

Ader, R. (1982). Behaviorally conditioned immunosuppression and murine system in Lupus erythematosus. *Science* 215:1534-1536.

Calden, G., Dupertius, C.W., Hokanson, J.E. & Lewis, W.M.C. (1960). Psychosomatic factors in the rate of recovery from tuberculosis. *Psychosom. Med.* 22:345-355.

Coe, C.L., Rosenberg, L.T., Fischer, M. & Levine, S. (1987). Psychological factors capable of preventing the inhibition of antibody responses in infant monkeys. *Child Dev.* 58(6):1420-1430.

Darko, D.F., Lucas, A.H., Gillin, J.C., Risch, S.C., Golshan, S., Hamburger, R.N., Silverman, M.B. & Janowsky, D.S. (1988). Cellular immunity and the hypothalamic-pituitary axis in major affective disorder. A preliminary study. *Psychiatry Res.* 25 (1):1-10.

Frerichs, F.T. (1858). Klinik der Leberkrankheiten, Erster Band. Vieweg, Braunschweig.

Ghanta, V.K., Hiramoto, R.N., Solvason, H.B. & Spector, N.H. (1985). Neural and environmental influences on neoplasia and conditioning of NK activity. *J. Immunol.* 135: 848-852.

Gidaly, M., Gorgan, V., Iepureanu, A., Sirbu, A. & Schuster, N. (1964). Neuro-psychische Erscheinungen bei der Hepatitis infectiosa. *Z. Ges. Inn. Medizin* 19:519-522.

Imboden, J.B., Canter, A. & Cluff, L.E. (1961). Convalescence from influenza. *Arch. Intern. Med.* 108:393-399.

Kasl, S.V., Evans, A.S. & Niederman, J.C. (1979). Psychosocial risk factors in the development of infectious mononucleosis. *Psychosom. Med.* 41:445-466.

Kennedy, S., Kiecolt-Glaser, J.K. & Glaser, R. (1988). Immunological consequences of acute and chronic stressors: Mediating role of interpersonal relationships. *Brit. J. Med. Psychol.* 61:77-85.

Kiecolt-Glaser, J.K., Glaser, R., Strain, E.C., Stout, J.C., Tarr, K.L., Holliday, J.E. & Speicher, C. (1986). Modulation of cellular immunity in medical students. *J. Behav. Med.* 9:5-21.

Kipshagen, H. (1975). *Psychische Veränderungen bei der akuten Virushepatitis in einer Verlaufsstudie mit dem MMPI-Saarbrücken-Persönlichkeitstest.* Dissertationsschrift München.

Laudenslager, M.I., Ryan, S.M., Drugan, R.C., Hyson, R.L. & Maier, S.F. (1983). Coping and immunosuppression: Inescapable but not escapable shock suppresses lymphocyte proliferation. *Science* 221:568-570.

Leibowitz, S. & Gorman, W.F. (1952). Neuropsychiatric complications of viral hepatitis. *N. Engl. J. Med.* 246:932-937.

Meyer zum Büschenfelde, K.H. (1987). Immunologie der Lebererkrankungen. *Schweiz. med. Wschr.* 117:1065-1075.

Paar, G.H., Schaefer, A. & Drexler, W. (1987). Über das Mitwirken psychosozialer Faktoren bei Ausbruch und Verlauf der akuten Virushepatitis - Bericht über eine Pilotstudie. *Psychother. Med. Psychol.* 37:23-30.

Schleifer, S.J., Keller, S.E., Siris, S.G., Davis, K.L. & Stein, M. (1985). Depression and immunity. Lymphocyte function in ambulatory depressed patients, hospitalized schizophrenic patients and patients hospitalized for herniorrhaphy. *Arch. Gen. Psychiat.* 42:129-133.

Solomon, G.F., Temoshok, L., O'Leary, A. & Zich, J. (1986). An intensive psycho-immunologic study of long-surviving persons with AIDS. Pilot work, background studies, hypotheses and methods. *Ann. NY Aca. Sci.* 496:756.

Zeichen, R. (1986). Vergleichende Untersuchung über die Persönlichkeitsstruktur des Diabetikers und des chronisch Leberkranken. *Wien Med. Wochenschr. (Suppl)* 96:1-12.

Chapter 17

Stress, Tumor Metastasis and Effectiveness of Antitumor Chemotherapy

Tullio Giraldi
Laura Perissin
Valentina Rapozzi
Sonia Zorzet

Institute of Pharmacology
University of Triest, Italy

Introduction

The notion that psychological factors can be related to tumor incidence and progression has been repeatedly put forward for clinical cancer (Rosch, 1984; Greer & Watson, 1987) and is confirmed by a considerable amount of experimental evidence. The application of stressor paradigms to laboratory animals resulted in modification of the growth of spontaneous and transplanted tumors, and several available reviews deal in detail with the results obtained (Steplewski et al., 1987; Vogel, 1987; Riley et al., 1981; LaBarba, 1970). It has to be noted, however, that rather conflicting evidence was obtained from these investigations in several instances, and tumor progression was found to be sometimes enhanced or decreased, or also left unaffected (Riley, 1979; Sklar & Anisman, 1981). It has been proposed that these discrepancies may be explained, at least partially, by the different nature of the stressors examined, by the timing of their application in relation to the phase of tumor growth, and by the acute or chronic administration of the stressors themselves (Justice, 1985). Moreover, the different investigations performed used widely differing tumor-host systems, including spontaneous tumors and tumors induced by carcinogens (viral, chemical and physical ones), or transplanted neoplasms; some of the tumors were solid, and sometimes ascitic or leukemic lines were used (Justice, 1985). The majority of tumor-host systems were allogeneic, and only a limited number of reports specifically studied the effects of stress on tumor metastasis, in spite of its clinical relevance. The interest of the potential effects of psychological stress on tumor metastasis is further indicated by unequivocal data, showing that the physical stress resulting from diagnostic and therapeutic procedures, such as radiotherapy (Van den Brenk & Kelly, 1973; Withers & Milas, 1973; Furuse & Kasuga, 1982; Peters, 1975), chemotherapy (de Ruiter et al., 1979; Orr et al, 1986; Ormerod et al., 1986), anaesthesia (Lundy et al., 1978) and surgery (Peters, 1975; Lundy et al., 1978; Agostino & Agostino, 1979; Pollock et al., 1984), increases metastasis formation in laboratory animals bearing malignant tumors.

Thus the aim of this contribution has been to illustrate the results obtained by examining the effects of the application of controlled paradigms of psychological stress on mice bearing a syngeneic solid malignant tumor which has spontaneously metastasized to the lungs, i.e. Lewis lung carcinoma. The stressor paradigms explored were also chosen considering their analogy to some factors which have been suggested to be of relevance in clinical psycho-oncological investigations (Greer & Watson, 1987; Temoshok, 1987). Housing in a low stress (protected) environment in comparison with a conventional animal room and the anxiety caused by periodic subjection of the animals kept in the protected environment to spatial disorientation, as originally devised by Riley et al. (1981),.were examined. The other stressors employed included maternal deprivation (LaBarba et al., 1970), physical restraint (Gotoh et al., 1986), behavioural despair (Porsolt et al., 1987), and avoidable vs. unavoidable foot shock in conditioned and non-conditioned animals (Sklar & Anisman, 1979). The effects of the application of these stressors on primary s.c. tumor growth and on the formation of spontaneous metastasis were examined differentially. In order to gain information on the neuro-endocrine mechanisms underlying the effects of psychological stress on tumor metastasis, direct hormonal assays were performed, and pharmacological inhibitors of nervous and endocrine functions were used *in vivo* . The hormones assayed were corticosterone in plasma and the urinary excretion of melatonin. To elucidate the role played by this hormone, different light-dark cycles effective in controlling pineal function were also used. The pharmacological agents tested *in vivo* included mitotane as an adrenal gland suppressor, naltrexone as an antagonist of β-endorphin, bromocryptine as a prolactin inhibitor, and the adrenolytic agents reserpine and guanethidine. The results obtained are reported later in this paper.

Materials and methods

Animals and tumor transplantation: The animals used were female C57BL/6 and C57BL/6 x DBA/2 F^1 (hereafter called BD2F1) mice weighing 18-20 g each, purchased from Charles River, Calco, Como, Italy. Lewis lung carcinoma was originally provided by the National Cancer Institute, Bethesda, MD, U.S.A., and was maintained in C57BL/6 mice by s.c. injection in the axillary region of 50 mm^3 of minced tumor tissue aseptically prepared from donors similarly inoculated two weeks earlier (Geran et al., 1972). For experimental purposes, the tumor was propagated in BD2F1 mice by s.c. injection of 10^6 tumor cells using a suspension of tumor cells prepared as already described (Sava et al., 1983).

Measurement of tumor growth and metastasis formation: Primary tumor weight (g) was determined 14 days after tumor inoculation by caliper measurements of short (a) and long (b) axes (cm), taking a tumor density equal to 1:

$$\text{Tumor weight} = \pi/6 \times a^2 \times b \qquad \text{(A)}$$

The number of metastases was determined at sacrifice on day 22 from tumor inoculation by examining the surface of the lungs with a low-power stereo-microscope. The weight of the metastases was determined as the sum of their individual weights calculated according to equation (A) after determination of their dimensions with an ocular micrometer (Sava et al., 1984).

Animal housing and spatial disorientation: The animals were kept 5 to a cage in order to avoid the effects of overcrowding or isolation on tumor progression (Riley et al., 1981; Labarba, 1970). The cages were placed in the protected environment for 2 weeks before tumor inoculation to allow the animals time to recover from the stress of shipment (Riley et al., 1981; LaBarba, 1970; Riley, Fitzmaurice et al., 1981) and to adapt them to the new housing conditions. The protected environment consisted of a cabinet with laminar air flow containing the animal cages, which minimized acoustic, olfactory and visual communication between the cages themselves and also with events outside of the cabinet (Riley et al., 1981). The cabinets were contained in a room set apart from the other animal rooms, where staff entered only once every 5 days to supply the animals with food and water which were given *ad libitum* . The light-dark cycle in the room was 12-12 hr, with an intensity in the cages of approximately 5 lux; when different light cycles were examined in relation to melatonin secretion, as indicated, light intensity in the cages was 2,100 lux. Constant temperature and relative humidity were 20°C and 60%, respectively.

The animals in the low-stress environment were subjected to spatial disorientation (rotational stress), when indicated, by spinning the cages at 45 rpm for 10 min every hour from the time of tumor inoculation until sacrifice (Riley et al., 1981).

Further stressor paradigms: In addition to examining the effects of housing conditions and of subjection to spatial disorientation, other stressor paradigms (physical restraint, behavioural despair, electric foot shock and maternal deprivation) were also employed. The stressors used are described below and were applied to mice housed both before and during the experiment in a partially protected environment, identical to that described above but omitting to maintain the cages in the protective cabinet.

Physical restraint consisted of placing mice individually into small opaque plastic tubes with a length of 10 cm and a diameter of 5 cm (permitting movement) or of 2.8 cm (not permitting movement). The animals remained in the tubes 2 hrs a day for 6 days following tumor inoculation.

Behavioural despair was induced by means of tail suspension, as performed in the test reported by Porsolt et al. (1987). The mice were hung individually in boxes from a hook, which allowed a distance of 15 cm from the walls, by an adhesive tape attached 2 cm from the extremity of the tail. This procedure was performed 10 min/day for 6 days following tumor inoculation.

Electric foot shock experiments were performed essentially as described by Sklar & Anisman (1979), with mice placed individually in shuttle boxes measuring 30 x 14 x 15 cm. The boxes were divided into two compartments by a wall with an opening which allowed the mouse to interrupt (or prevent) the shock by moving to the opposite compartment. A light and sound warning lasting 5 sec preceded the beginning of the electric shock (1 mA) which was delivered through the grid floor and lasted 5 sec if uninterrupted. Sessions, consisting of the repetition of this cycle every 10 min for 3 hr, were repeated daily for 21 days following tumor inoculation. When indicated, animals conditioned before tumor inoculation to prevent the foot shock were used, which were chosen after 5 days of training by the above-described sessions. Conditioned and non-conditioned animals were also subjected to sessions of unavoidable foot shock after tumor transplantation, as indicated.

Maternal deprivation was induced by weaning at 14 days in contrast to separation at 21 days; five pups of the same sex were kept together in individual boxes. Special care was taken with feeding the pups, and tumor implantation was performed at 45 days of age (LaBarba et al., 1971).

Hormonal assays: The corticosterone levels in plasma were assayed fluorimetrically, as described by Nicholson & Peytremann (1975). Blood samples were obtained by intracardiac puncture of the animals immediately after sacrifice at 9 a.m.; blood collection required less than 1 min per mouse and was performed on one mouse at a time in a separate room in order to avoid influences on the animals awaiting sacrifice.

The urinary melatonin excretion was measured by means of a radioimmunoassay. The mice were housed individually for 24 hr during urine collection, and urine was recovered on Whatman 3MM filter paper placed under the stainless steel grid floor. Melatonin was eluted by washing the filter paper twice in 0.07 M phosphate buffer pH 5.5. This eluate was purified in a single chromatographic step using a C-18 column (Sep-Pak Water Associates, Millipore) to remove unknown materials which would interfere with subsequent RIA assay. The fraction obtained with chloroform as eluant was evaporated under a stream of nitrogen, and the melatonin present in this fraction was assayed by a ^{125}I radioimmunoassay (Clone-system Diagnostics, Nuclear Medica, Padova, Italy). Appropriate blanks were run, and recovery of melatonin from the urine using this method was 93% (± 5) in the range 20-320 pg/ml.

Drug treatment: Cyclophosphamide was kindly provided by Shering S.p.A., Milan, Italy. Mitotane and naltrexone were generously provided by the National Cancer Institute, Drug Synthesis and Chemistry Branch, Bethesda, U.S.A. and by Du Pont Pharmaceuticals, R & D, Geneva, Switzerland, respectively. Guanethidine and reserpine were kindly supplied by Ciba-Geigy S.p.A., Origgio, Varese, Italy. Bromocryptine was donated by Sandoz Prodotti Farmaceutici S.p.A., Milano, Italy. The drugs were administered p.o. on days 1-21 from tumor implantation and were admixed in powdered food (Altromin-R, supplied by A. Rieper S.p.A., Vandoies, Bolzano, Italy) in the concentration required for daily administration of the dosage indicated in the tables, with a measured daily food consumption of 5.0 ± 0.1 g per mouse.

Results

Effects of animal housing, spatial disorientation and other stressors: Representative results obtained by examining the effects of housing conditions and spatial disorientation on primary tumor growth and spontaneous lung metastasis formation in mice bearing Lewis lung carcinoma are presented in Table 1 which has been prepared, with minor modifications, from Giraldi et. al. (in press); replication of the experiment on three further occasions provided substantially identical results. When the tumor was implanted into mice, adapted before tumor implantation and further maintained afterward in the protected environment, the weight of spontaneous pulmonary metastases was significantly and markedly reduced in comparison with mice kept in conventional housing for the whole duration of the experiment. The subjection of animals kept continuously in the protected housing to a controlled paradigm of psychological stress (spatial disorientation) before and after tumor implantation significantly and markedly increased the number and weight of pulmonary metastases. There were no statistically significant differences ($p < 0.05$) between the values obtained for mice kept continuously in conventional housing and those for mice placed in the protected environment after tumor implantation and eventually subjected to spatial disorientation. The handling of mice, kept constantly in the protected environment, for the daily intraperitoneal administration of physiological saline significantly increased the weight and number of lung metastases to a value not significantly different ($p < 0.05$) from that observed after subjection to spatial disorientation. The effects of handling for the daily intraperitoneal administration of saline were not cumulative with those of spatial disorientation upon animals kept in the protected environment, nor were they significant in the other experimental groups, including animals kept constantly in the conventional housing. A statistically significant increase in primary tumor growth was observed in the group of animals kept continuously in the protected environment and subjected to spatial disorientation as compared with the other experimental groups. This increase was also maintained when handling was combined with spatial disorientation.

Treatment with cyclophosphamide per os on days 1-6 from tumor implantation was curative in 10/10 animals kept in the protected environment; the subjection of these animals to spatial disorientation reduced the cure rate to 0/10, with a significant reduction in primary tumor growth and metastases number and weight. Substantially identical results were obtained when the experiment was repeated a further three times, and representative results are illustrated in Table 2 which has been prepared, with minor modifications, from Giraldi et al. (1989).

The effects of the other stressors were examined by applying the paradigms used to animals maintained in the partially protected environment. Maternal deprivation, consisting of early

Table 1. Effects of housing conditions, spatial disorientation and handling for parenteral saline administration on primary tumor growth and spontaneous lung metastasis formation in mice bearing Lewis lung carcinoma.

SD (DAYS)	HOUSING BEFORE TUMOR INOCULATION	HOUSING AFTER TUMOR INOCULATION	INTRAPERITONEAL SALINE ADMINISTRATION	TUMOR WEIGHT (g)	METASTASIS NUMBER	METASTASIS WEIGHT (mg)
-	CONVENTIONAL	CONVENTIONAL	-	1.6±0.2♥•	44.2±5.8*♦	220.2± 61.6*
-	"	"	+	1.9±0.2♥•	47.3±7.6*♦	205.3± 30.1*
-	CONVENTIONAL	PROTECTED	-	1.8±0.3♥•	60.2±1.3*	354.2± 123.4*
-	"	"	+	1.4±0.1♥•	54.0±11.0	332.4± 72.4*
0-6	"	"	-	1.7±0.5♥•	47.8±11.8	266-0± 122.0*
0-6	"	"	+	2.1±0.4♥•	68.7±16.0*	255.7± 106.5*
-	PROTECTED	PROTECTED	-	2.0±0.3#	32.6±6.7#	70.7± 25.6#
-	"	"	+	2.0±0.4♥	57.8±9.0*	278.0± 76.7*
0-6	"	"	-	4.0±1.7*♣	80.5±7.0*♠	281.2± 80.8*
0-6	"	"	+	3.7±1.2*o	59.0±8.8*	223.0± 44.8*

Spatial disorientation (SD) was applied to mice in the protected housing for 7 (0-6) days from tumor inoculation. Each value is the mean (±SE) obtained using groups of 5 mice. When indicated, the animals received i.p. on days 1-21 0.1 ml of isotonic NaCl solution (9 g/l). t-test for grouped data (52) $p < 0.05$; *: means significantly different from #: ♥: means significantly different from ♣; •: means significantly different from o and ♦: means significantly different from ♠.

Tab. 2: Primary tumor growth and spontaneous lung metastasis formation in mice bearing Lewis lung carcinoma cept in protected housing, subjected to spatial disorientation (SD) and treated with cyclophosphamide.

SD	TREATMENT WITH CY	PRIMARY TUMOR WEIGHT (g)	METASTASES NUMBER	METASTASES WEIGHT (mg)	METASTASES FREE
-	-	2.1 ± 0.5[a*]	41 ± 6[c*]	127 ± 19[e*]	0/10
-	+	-	-	-	10/10
+	-	3.4 ± 0.3[a*, b*]	60 ± 5[c*, d*]	189 ± 14[e*, f**]	0/10
+	+	1.1 ± 0.3[b**]	13 ± 2[d**]	26 ± 4[f**]	0/10

Each value is the mean (± SE) obtained using groups of 10 mice treated, as indicated, with cyclophosphamide (CY, 240 mg/kg/day) on days 1-6 from tumor inoculation.
: means with the same letter are significantly different, t-test for grouped data, (: $p < 0.05$; **: $p < 0.01$).

Tab. 3: Effects of maternal deprivation on primary tumor growth and spontaneous loung metastasis formation in mice bearing Lewis lung carcinoma.

TIME OF WEANING (DAYS)	SEX	PRIMARY TUMOR GROWTH (g)	METASTASES NUMBER	METASTASES WEIGHT (mg)
14	FEMALE	5.1 ± 0.3	30 ± 5	125 ± 26*
21	FEMALE	5.4 ± 0.4	45 ± 3	236 ± 28*
14	MALE	5.5 ± 0.4	35 ± 5	127 ± 21
21	MALE	6.0 ± 0.5	39 ± 4	147 ± 36

Each value is the mean (± SE) obtained using groups of 6-14 C57/B16 mice, which were separated from their mothers when indicated.

*: means statistically different; t-test for grouped data.

weaning at 14 days, was devoid of significant effects in male mice; in female mice maternal separation caused a significant decrease in lung metastasis weight (Table 3). Limited physical restraint, produced by placing the animals individually into relatively large plastic tubes, was devoid of significant effects when compared with non-stressed controls, whereas more severe restraint significantly increased the number and weight of lung metastases. On the other hand, behavioural despair induced by tail suspension significantly increased primary tumor growth and decreased the number and weight of pulmonary metastases in the same animals (Table 4). When the effects of applying foot shock were examined, a high variability was observed. A tendency toward an increase in tumor growth and metastasis formation appeared in non-conditioned mice subjected to avoidable foot shock; a significant decrease in metastasis number, accompanied by a non-significant decrease in metastasis weight and increase in primary tumor weight, was observed in preconditioned mice subjected to sessions of avoidable foot shock after tumor implantation (Table 5).

Plasmatic corticosterone and effects of mitotane: The subjection of animals kept in the protected environment to spatial disorientation caused a significant increase in the plasmatic level of corticosterone, which accompanied the significant increase in metastasis weight and number. When the animals were treated with mitotane, the drug did not modify the base level of corticosterone but totally abolished the increase produced by spatial disorientation. In spite of these inhibitory effects on the corticosterone level, the increase in lung metastasis formation caused by spatial disorientation was maintained in mice treated with mitotane (Table 6) (Perissin et al., 1989).

Effects of treatment with pharmacological inhibitors of neuro-vegetative and endocrine functions on tumor growth and metastasis: The effects of treatment with the tested drugs were determined in mice kept in the protected environment and subjected to spatial disorientation. None of the tested drugs significantly modified primary tumor growth, and naltrexone was also devoid of effects on metastasis. On the contrary, a significant reduction in the number and weight of lung metastases was produced by the other drugs, which was remarkably pronounced for reserpine (Table 7).

Urinary melatonin excretion in relation to tumor growth and metastasis: When different cycles of illumination with an intensity of 2,100 lux were used, the effects of subjection to spatial disorientation consisted in a significant reduction in the weight of lung metastases accompanied by a non-significant influence on primary tumor growth and metastasis number. This reduction was more pronounced for constant lighting and contrasted with the results presented in Table 1, which were obtained with a light-dark cycle of 12/12 hr and an intensity of 5 lux. The nocturnal

Tab. 4: Effects of physical restraint and behavioral despair on primary tumor growth and spontaneous lung metastasis formation in mice bearing Lewis lung carcinoma.

STRESS	PRIMARY TUMOR GROWTH (g)	METASTASIS	
		NUMBER	WEIGHT (mg)
-	2.4 ± 0.5	31 ± 6	135 ± 34
PRPM[a]	1.7 ± 0.3	33 ± 2	186 ± 23
PRNPM[b]	1.6 ± 0.1	51 ± 7*	272 ± 38*
BD[c]	2.6 ± 0.3	28 ± 5	108 ± 19

a: physical restraint permitting movement;
b: physical restraint not permitting movement;
c: behavioural despair

Each value is the mean (± SE) obtained using groups of 10 mice subjected to the indicated stressor paradigms.
*: means statistically different from the relevant controls, t-test for grouped data (52), $p < 0.05$.

Tab. 5: Effects of avoidable foot-shock on primary tumor growth and spontaneous lung metastasis formation in pre-conditioned mice or non-conditioned mice bearing Lewis lung carcinoma.

FOOT-SHOCK	PRIMARY TUMOR GROWTH (g)	METASTASIS	
		NUMBER	WEIGHT (mg)
-	2.0 ± 0.3	15 ± 1	59 ± 17
+#	2.9 ± 0.3	10 ± 1*	27 ± 8
+@	2.8 ± 0.2	21 ± 5	104 ± 39

Each value is the mean (± SE) obtained using groups of 5 pre-conditioned (#) or non-conditioned (@) mice exposed to avoidable foot s hock, as indicated.

*: mean statistically different from the relevant control, t-test for grouped data (52), $p < 0.05$

Table 6. Effects of mitotane on plasma corticosterone, primary tumor growth and spontaneous lung metastasis formation in mice bearing Lewis lung carcinoma.

SD	HOUSING	MITOTANE	PLASMA CORTICOSTERONE (ng/ml)	TUMOR WEIGHT	METASTASIS	
					NUMBER	WEIGHT (mg)
-	PROTECTED	-	96.4 ± 2.8	2.3 ± 0.2	19.4 ± 1.8	61.6 ± 8.6
-	PROTECTED	+	103.4 ± 13.7	1.5 ± 0.3	21.4 ± 3.6	61.8 ± 16.0
+	PROTECTED	-	252.8 ± 3.4*	3.5 ± 0.4*	29.7 ± 1.6*	135.1 ± 12.8*
+	PROTECTED	+	101.5 ± 10.3	3.1 ± 0.4	32.4 ± 8.1*	131.6 ± 29.9*

Each value is the mean (± SE) obtained using groups of 10 mice.
*: means significantly different from that of untreated controls without spatial disorientation (SD), t-test for grouped data (52), $p < 0.05$.

Tab. 7: Effects of treatment with pharmacological inhibitors of neurovegetative and endocrine functions on primary tumor growth and spontaneous lung metastasis formation in mice bearing Lewis lung carcinoma subjected to spatial disorientation.

TREATMENT	DOSE (mg/kg/day)	PRIMARY TUMOR GROWTH (g)	METASTASIS	
			NUMBER	WEIGHT (mg)
GUANETHIDINE	60	60 ± 3	36 ± 25*	28 ± 5*
RESERPINE	2.5	65 ± 12	19 ± 5*	9 ± 3*
NALTREXONE	8	121 ± 29	53 ± 6	40 ± 7
BROMOCRYPTINE	10	65 ± 1	37 ± 6*	32 ± 6*

Each value is the mean (± SE) per cent ratio obtained using groups of 10 drug-treated mice as compaired with drug untreated controls.
*: mean different from that of drug-untreated controls, t-test for grouped data, p<0.05

urinary excretion of melatonin was consistently higher than that determined during light hours with the three light cycles examined; nocturnal melatonin levels were markedly and significantly increased by subjecting the animals to spatial disorientation when they were kept under constant illumination (Table 8) (Persissin et al., in press).

Discussion

A relatively large number of reports exist in the literature showing that stress can influence the incidence and progression of tumors in laboratory animals (Steplewski et al., 1987; Vogel, 1987; Riley et al., 1981; LaBarba, 1970; Riley, 1979; Sklar & Anisman, 1981; Justice, 1985). The data available indicate that the physical stress produced by therapeutic procedures increases tumor metastasis in experimental animal-tumor systems. Psychological stressors, including isolation or overcrowding during animal housing, have also been shown to influence the

Table 8. Effects of different light cycles and spatial disorientation (SD) on urinary secretion of melatonin and primary tumor growth and spontaneous lung metastasis formation in mice bearing Lewis lung carcinoma.

SD	LIGHT/ DARK CYCLES	URINARY MELATONIN EXCRETION (pg) LIGHT	DARK	TUMOR WEIGHT (g)	METASTASIS NUMBER	WEIGHT (mg)
-	16/8	5.3 ± 1.6	48.9 ± 18.0♥	2.7 ± 0.2	39.4 ± 4.9	210.4 ± 27.4♠
+	16/8	6.4 ± 1.3	76.0 ± 5.0♥	3.0 ± 0.2	35.6 ± 3.1	150.5 ± 20.5
–	12/12	6.4 ± 2.4	68.9 ± 17.0♥	3.6 ± 0.3	36.9 ± 4.4	167.4 ± 26.4
+	12/12	6.0 ± 2.1	92.0 ± 21.0♥	3.2 ± 0.4	26.4 ± 2.9	107.4 ± 9.8♦•
–	24/0	6.6 ± 1.5@	46.8 ± 15.3&♥	3.1 ± 0.3	44.8 ± 5.7	219.1 ± 37.7o
+	24/0	6.8 ± 2.1@	152.0 ± 20.0&♣	2.8 ± 0.3	29.1 ± 5.2	95.1 ± 22.4♦•

Each value is the mean (± SE) obtained using groups of 10 mice. Melatonin was determined on day 15 @: 8 a.m. - 8 p.m.; &: 8 p.m. - 8.a.m.). Student-Neumann-Keuls test (52), $p < 0.05$, ♥: means significantly different from ♣; ♦: means significantly different from ♠: • means significantly different from o.

incidence and growth of tumors in laboratory rodents (Steplewski et al., 1987; Riley et al., 1981; LaBarba, 1970). The results obtained with psychological stressors are rather conflicting and appear to depend on the experimental conditions chosen, i.e. the animal-tumor system used, the acute or chronic application of the stressor, as well as its nature (Justice, 1985). Moreover, the majority of the animal-tumor systems employed in these studies were allogeneic, and metastasis was rarely examined (Justice, 1985) in spite of the clinical relevance of this phenomenon.

An absolute distinction between physical and psychological stressors appears to be difficult; for instance, a certain degree of subjective cognitive and emotional reaction is presumably always present when coping with physical stressors. In the present investigation the first series of stressor variables examined were housing conditions, handling the animals for intraperitoneal drug administration, and periodic subjection to spatial disorientation. These stressors appeared mainly to be of a psychological nature, and spatial disorientation, in particular, was suggested to be an emotional stressor (anxiety) (Riley et al., 1981,a), since the centrifugal acceleration produced in the cages by rotation was smaller than 0.15 g. Using these conditions, with a light-dark cycle of 12-12 hr, an intensity of 5 lux in the cages and Lewis lung carcinoma implanted into syngeneic BD2F1 mice as the animal-tumor system, the results reported show that tumor metastasis is reduced independently of primary tumor growth by housing the animals in a low-stress environment. Subjection to spatial disorientation and the handling of animals for intraperitoneal administration of physiological saline increases metastasis number and weight and primary tumor growth in animals kept in the low-stress housing. This increase is not cumulative when spatial disorientation and handling are combined and is not observed when the mice are not adapted before and kept after tumor implantation in the low-stress housing. The tumor responses presently caused by housing conditions, handling and spatial disorientation are of a similar magnitude; their observed non-cumulative action might depend on the fact that each of them represents the maximal degree of control exerted by the host in response to the stressors applied. This interpretation is consistent with the data obtained in several other studies, which show that in certain circumstances the effect of one stressor can be non-cumulative with, modified by, and even reverted by the combined application of further stressors, depending on their nature and the timing of application (Riley, 1979; Sklar & Anisman, 1981). This view is further supported by the (unreported) results obtained when spatial disorientation was combined with surgery, which indicated that the effects of spatial disorientation were reverted by surgery, leading to a reduction in tumor metastasis.

When cyclophosphamide is administered to mice in the protected environment, all of the treated mice are cured; the subjection of these animals to spatial disorientation totally abolishes the curative action of the drug. The treatment with cyclophosphamide, as well as all of the other *in vivo* pharmacological treatment performed for the experiments reported in this work, was carried out orally by admixing the drug with powdered food in order to eliminate the significant influence of handling the animals for parenteral administrations, illustrated above. It is noteworthy that spatial disorientation abolishes the curative action of cyclophosphamide in animals receiving the drug at a dosage and on a schedule that strongly depresses T-cell-dependent and NK-mediated immune responses (Hilgard et al., 1985; Mantovani et al., 1977). This finding is consistent with the results obtained in similar conditions with ICRF159, since the reduction of metastasis formation by this drug with a non-cytotoxic mechanism is reduced upon subjecting the treated animals to spatial disorientation (Giraldi et al., 1988).

The results obtained by examining the other stressor paradigms tested in animals kept in the partially protected housing are preliminary; they present a relatively high variability, and it has not yet been determined whether this is intrinsic for the experimental conditions employed or further controllable. The general conclusions that can be drawn at present are limited and indicate that these stressors influence tumor spread, either increasing or decreasing spontaneous metastasis in a way which is independent of the effects on primary tumor growth. These results add meaningful information to that contained in available reports on the effects of maternal deprivation, foot shock and physical restraint, which were examined only in relation to primary tumor growth and mainly using allogeneic animal-tumor systems (Justice, 1985).

From the results presented above it might be interpreted that, because the central nervous system modulates natural antitumor responses of the host via neural vegetative and endocrine mechanisms (Riley et al., 1982), coping with stressors may lead to a reduction in these responses (Borisenko & Borisenko, 1982; Borisenko & Kandil, 1985). Consequently, during the present investigation an examination was performed to determine the significance of some of the mediating mechanisms among the numerous ones which have been suggested in general to mediate the effects of stress on tumor progression (Borisenko & Borisenko, 1982; Borisenko, 1982). The evidence presented allows us to rule out a significant participation of corticosterone in the experimental conditions used. This conclusion is further supported by the reported observation that the antimetastatic action of ICRF159 is not modified when treatment with this drug is combined with mitotane (Giraldi et al., 1988). β-endorphin similarly appears to have a marginal role, as indicated by the ineffectiveness of the *in vivo* treatment of tumor-bearing mice with naltrexone, at dosages capable of antagonizing *in vivo* the analgesic effects of morphine in mice (Zagon & McLaughlin, 1987). The significant effects on metastasis of treatment with bromocryptine, at dosages effective in maintaining the plasmatic prolactin at levels similar to those of hypophysiectomized mice (Rao et al., 1984), suggest a substantial participation of prolactin. Finally, the adrenergic system appears to play a significant role in the modulation of tumor metastasis by spatial disorientation, as indicated by the remarkable inhibition caused by reserpine and guanethidine. The effectiveness of both drugs indicates that central and peripheral adrenergic mechanisms are involved; for reserpine, sedation can be excluded as the cause of the reported effects, since treatment with barbiturates at sedative dosages is ineffective (unreported results).

Numerous biological functions have been found to implicate the pineal gland and melatonin (Axelrod, 1974); as far as neoplasms are concerned, pineal function and melatonin secretion have been related to the control of tumor growth (Lissoni et al., 1987), immune function (Jancovic et al., 1970) and stress responses (Pierpaoli & Maestroni, 1987), in general, and to the process of tumor metastasis, in particular (Barone & Das Gupta, 1970; Lapin, 1974, 1975). The results presented indeed indicate that pineal function is involved in tumor metastasis and its modulation by stress. In fact, different intensities of illumination with constant light-dark cycles, and different light-dark cycles with the same intensity of illumination significantly influence metastasis formation. This finding is in agreement with the already reported effects of different light cycles, which were limited to primary tumor growth only (Riley, 1979) and to the use of modifications of light cycles considered as an experimental stressor (Kort et al., 1986). Urinary excretion of melatonin is increased by stress in mice under intense illumination, and this increase is associated with a reduction in metastasis formation. The complexity of the central neurochemical mechanisms governing pineal function and melatonin increase and the ambiguity of its peripheral targets and actions (Brown & Niles, 1982) make further interpretation of the results illustrated difficult at this stage of research.

In conclusion, the experimental results presented indicate that psychological stressors can influence tumor metastasis in mice bearing a syngeneic solid malignant tumor in a way which is independent of the effects on primary tumor growth; the mediation of multiple neuroendocrine mechanisms has been preliminarily identified. The finding that the effectiveness of antitumor chemotherapy is dramatically reduced by a psychological stressor appears noteworthy. Moreover, the results presented support the possibility previously indicated by Riley that pharmacological agents can be used in order to inhibit hosts' responses to applied stressors (Riley, 1979). Further research is needed, and is partially in progress, aiming to identify and characterize further the neuroendocrine and immunological mediators of the responses to the stressors presently used; the actual data seem, however, of interest for their experimental and clinical implications.

Acknowledgements: This work is supported by the Italian National Research Couuncil, Special Project 'Oncology' contract no 88.00691.44, and by grants from the Ministry of Education (MPI 40 and 60%). The outstanding technical assistance of Mr. G. Fonzari is recognized, and the generosity of Fondazione C. & D. Callerio in providing the protected animal rooms is gratefully appreciated.

References

Agostino, D. & Agostino, N. (1979). Role of operative trauma: explosive metastasis of similar size following amputation of the primary leg tumor. *Tumori* 65:527.

Axelrod, J. (1974). The pineal gland: a neurochemical transducer. *Science* 184:1341.

Barone, R.M. & Das Gupta, T.K. (1970). Role of pinealectomy in Walker 256 carcinoma in rats. *J. Surg. Oncol.* 2:313.

Borisenko, J.Z. (1982). Higher cortical function and neoplasia: psychoneuroimmunology. In: Levy, S.M.(Ed.). *Biological mediators of behaviour and disease: neoplasia.* Elsevier Biomedical, New York, 29.

Borisenko, M. & Borisenko, J.Z. (1982). Stress behavior and immunity: animal models and mediating mechanisms. Gen. Hosp. *Psychiatry* 4:59.

Borisenko, M. & Kandil, O. (1985). Stress-induced decline in natural killer cell activity, cytotoxic cell function and interleukin-2 production. Relationship with tumor growth in C3H/HeJ mice. In: Bennett, C.B. (Ed.). *Neuroimmunomodulation. Proceedings of the First International Workshop on Neuroimmunomodulation, Bethesda.* Published by the International Working Group on Neuroimmunomodulation, 262.

Brown, G.M. & Niles, L.P. (1982). Studies on melatonin and other pineal factors. In: Besser, G.M. & Martini, L. (Eds.) *Clinical neuroendocrinology.* Academic Press, New York, Vol. 2, 205.

de Ruiter, J., Cramer, S.J., Smink, T. & van Putten, L.M. (1979). The facilisation of tumor growth in the lung by cyclophosphamide in artificial and spontaneous metastase model. *Eur. J. Cancer Clin. Oncol.* 15:1139.

Furuse, T. & Kasuga, T. (1982). Effects of irradiation with fast neutrons on X-rays on the incidence of metastasis of transplanted B16 melanoma in mice. *Gann* 73:35.

Geran, R.I., Greenberg, N.H., MacDonald, M.M., Schumacher, A.M. & Abbott, B.J. (1972). Abbott BJ. Protocols for screening chemical agents and natural products against animal tumors and other biological systems. *Cancer Chemother. Rep*. 3:13.

Giraldi, T., Perissin, L., Piccini, P., Rapozzi, V. & Zorzet, S. (1989). Stress, tumor progression and success of chemotherapy in mice. In: Hadden, J.W., Masek, K. & Nisticò, G. (Eds.). *Interactions among CNS, neuroendocrine and immune systems*. Pythagora Press, Rome-Milan, 429.

Giraldi, T., Perissin, L., Sava, G., Zorzet, S., Nicpali, S. & Rodani, M.G. (1988). Is effectiveness of cancer chemotherapy influenced by stress? In: Lobo, A. & Tres, A. (Eds.). *Psicosomatica y cancer*. Graficas Solana, Madrid, 73.

Giraldi, T., Perissin, L., Zorzet, S., Piccini, P. & Rapozzi, V. Effects of stress on tumor growth and metastasis in mice bearing Lewis lung carcinoma. *Eur. J.. Cancer Clin. Oncol.* (in press).

Gotoh, T., Ganhon, L. & Yoshikura, H. (1986). Effects of physical restraint on leukemogenesis by friend virus. *Gann* 77:985.

Greer, S.G. & Watson, M. (1987). Mental adjustment to cancer: its measurement and prognostic importance. *Cancer Surveys* 6:439.

Hilgard, P., Phol, J., Steckar, J. & Voegeli, R. (1985). Oxaphosphorines as biological response modifiers - experimental and clinical perspectives. *Cancer Treat. Rev.* 12:155.

Jankovic, B.D., Isakovic, K. & Petrovic, S. (1970). Effects of pinealectomy on immune reactions in the rat. *Immunology* 18:1.

Justice, A. (1985). Review of the effect of stress on cancer in laboratory animals: importance of time of stress application and type of tumor. *Psychol. Bull.* 98:108.

Kort, W.J., Zondervan, P.E., Hulsman, L.O.M., Weijma, I.M. & Westbroek, D.L. (1986). Light-darkshift stress with special reference to spontaneous tumor incidence in female BN rats. *JNCI* 76:439.

LaBarba, R.C. (1970). Experimental and environmental factors in cancer. *Psychosom. Med.* 32:258.

LaBarba, R.C., White, J.L., Lazar, J. & Klein, M. (1970). Early maternal separation and the response to early Ehrlich carcinoma in Balb/C mice. *Develop. Psychol.* 3:78.

Lapin, V. (1974). Influence of simultaneous thymectomy and pinealectomy on the growth and formation of metastasis of the Yoshida sarcoma in rats. *Exp. Pathol.* Jena 9:108.

Lapin, V. (1975). The pineal and neoplasia. *Lancet* 1:341.

Lissoni, P., Barni, S., Tancini, G., Crispino, S., Paolorossi, F., Lucini, V., Mariani, M., Cattaneo, G., Esposti, D., Esposti, G. & Fraschini, F. (1987). Chemical study of melatonin in untreatable advanced cancer patients. *Tumori* 73:475.

Lundy, J., Lowett, E.J., Hamilton, S. & Conran, P. (1978). Halothane, surgery, immune suppression and artificial pulmonary metastases. *Cancer* 41:827.

Mantovani, A., Polentarutti, N., Alessandri, G., Vecchi, A., Giuliani, F. & Spreafico, F. (1977). Activation of K-cells in mice with transplanted tumors differing in immunogenicity and metastasizing capacity. *Br. J. Cancer* 36:453.

Nicholson, W.E. & Peytremann, A. (1975). The rat adrenal in situ . *Meth. Enzymol.* 32:336.

Ormerod, E.J., Everett, C.A. & Hart, I.R. (1986). Enhanced experimental metastatic capacity of a human tumor line following treatment with 5-azacytidine. *Cancer Res.* 46:884.

Orr, F.W., Adamson, I.J.R. & Young, L. (1986). Promotion of pulmonary metasis in mice by bleomycin-induced endothelial injury. *Cancer Res.* 46:891.

Perissin, L., Zorzet, S., Piccini, P., Rapozzi, V. & Giraldi, T. (1989). Corticosterone does not mediate the effects of stress on tumor metastasis. *Pharmacol Res.* 21:461.

Perissin, L., Zorzet, S., Rapozzi V. & Giraldi, T. Effects of the different light cycles and stress on urinary excretion of melatonin and tumor spread in mice bearing Lewis lung carcinoma. *Pharmacol. Res.* (in press).

Peters, L.J. (1975). A study of the influence of various diagnostic and therapeutic procedures applied to a murine squamos carcinoma on its metastasic behavior. *Br. J. Cancer* 32:355.

Pierpaoli, W. & Maestroni, G.J.M. (1987). Melatonin: a principle neuroimmunregulatory and anti-stress hormone: its anti-aging effects. *Immunol. Lett.* 16:355.

Pollock, R.E., Babacock, G.F., Ronsdahl, M.M. & Mishioka, K. (1984). Surgical stress-mediated suppression of murine natural killer cell cytotoxity. *Cancer Res.* 44: 3888.

Porsolt, R.D., Chermat, R., Lenegre, A., Avril, I., Janvier, S. & Steru, L. (1987). Use of the automated tail suspension test for the primary screening psychotropic agents. *Arch. Int. Pharmacodyn* 288:11.

Rao, M.R., Bartke, A., Parkening, T.A. & Collins, T.J. (1984). Effect of treatment with different doses of bromocriptine on plasma profiles of prolactin, gonadotropins and testosterone in mature male rats and mice. *Int. J. Androl.* 7:258.

Riley, V. (1979). Cancer and stress, overview and critiue. *Cancer Detect. Prev.* 2:163.

Riley, V., Fitzmaurice, M.A. & Spackman, D.H. (1981,a). Animal models in biobehavioral research: effects of anxiety stress on immunocompetence and neoplasia. In: Weiss, S.M., Herd, J.A. & Fox, B.H. (Eds.). *Perspectives on behavioral medicine*. Academic Press, New York, 371.

Riley, V., Fitzmaurice, M.A. & Spackman, D.H. (1981). Psychoneuroimmunologic factors in neoplasia: studies in animals. In: Ader, R. (Ed.) *Psychoneuroimmunology*. Academic Press, New York, 31.

Riley, V., Fitzmaurice, M.A. & Spackman, H. (1982). Immunecompetence and neoplasia: role of anxiety stress. In: Levy S.M.(Ed.). *Biological mediators of behavior and disease: neoplasia.* Elsevier Biomedical, New York, 175.

Rosch, P.J. (1984). Stress and cancer. In: Cooper, C.L. (Ed.). *Psychosocial stress and cancer.* Chichester, John Wiley & Sons Ltd., 3.

Sava, G., Giraldi, T., Lassiani, L. & Dogani, R. (1983). Effects of isomeric aryldimethyltriazenes on Lewis lung carcinoma growth and metastasis in mice. *Chem. Biol. Interactions* 46:131.

Sava, G., Giraldi, T., Zupi, G. & Sacchi, A. (1984). Effects of antimetastatic dimethyltriazenes in mice bearing Lewis lung carcinoma lines with different metastatic potential. *Invasion metastasis* 4:171-178.

Sklar, L.S. & Anisman, H. (1979). Stress and coping factors influence tumor growth. *Science* 205:513.

Sklar, L.S. & Anisman, H. (1981). Stress and cancer. *Psychol. Bull.* 89:369.

Steplewski, Z., Robinson Goldman, P. & Vogel, W.H. (1987). Effects of housing stress on the formation and development of tumors in rats. *Cancer Letters* 34:257.

Tallarida, R.J. & Murray, R.B. (1987). *Manual of pharmacologic calculation with computer programs.* Springer-Verlag, New York.

Temoshok, L. (1987). Personality, coping style, emotion and cancer: towards an integrative model. *Cancer Surveys* 6:545.

Van den Brenk, H.A.S. & Kelly, H. (1973). Stimulation of growth of metastasis by local X-irradiation in kidney and liver. *Br. J. Cancer* 28:349.

Vogel, W.H. (1987). Stress neglected variable in experimental pharmacology and toxicology. *Trends Pharmacol. Sci.* 8:35.

Withers, H.R. & Milas, L. (1973). Influence of preirradiation of lung on development of artificial pulmonary metastases of fibrosarcoma in mice. *Cancer Res.* 33:1931.

Zagon, I.S. & McLaughlin, P.J. (1987). Modulation of murine neuroblastoma in nude mice by opioid antagonists. *JNCI* 78:141.

Chapter 18

Anticipatory Nausea and Immune Suppression in Cancer Patients Receiving Cycles of Chemotherapy: Conditioned Responses?

Dana H. Bovbjerg
William H. Redd

Psychoneuroimmunology Laboratory
Psychiatry Service
Memorial Sloan-Kettering Cancer Center, New York U.S.A.

Introduction

Animal studies have demonstrated that the immune system can be modulated by classical conditioning (Ader & Cohen, 1991). In their original experiment, Ader & Cohen (1991) found that rats could be conditioned by pairing the consumption of saccharin-flavored water (the conditioned stimulus) with an injection of cyclophosphamide (the unconditioned stimulus). When these conditioned animals were later re-exposed to the saccharin and challenged with antigen, they showed two conditioned responses - an aversion to the taste of saccharin and a reduction in serum antibody levels to the challenge antigen. Taste aversion per se was not responsible for the immune suppression since control rats conditioned with LiCl showed identical levels of taste aversion without any immune suppression. Subsequent experiments by several different laboratories have documented cyclophosphamide-induced conditioned suppression of a number of humoral and cell-mediated immune responses including plaque-forming cell responses; graft-vs-host responses; adjuvant induced arthritis; spleen cell mitogen responses; and natural killer (NK) cell activity (Ader & Cohen, 1991).

The human research that most closely parallels the study of conditioned effects induced by cyclophosphamide in animals is the analysis of anticipatory nausea and vomiting (ANV) in chemotherapy patients (Redd, 1989). After as few as two infusions, some patients become nauseated and vomit as they approach the hospital, upon seeing their doctor, or as a staff member prepares the infusion. Published estimates of the prevalence of ANV among chemotherapy patients (even those receiving antiemetic drugs) have ranged from 25% to 65%, depending upon the chemotherapy protocol (Carey & Burish, 1989; Morrow & Dobkin, 1989).

Research conducted to date is consistent with the hypothesis that ANV is the result of classical conditioning (Redd, 1989). According to this explanation ANV develops as a result of the repeated pairings of neutral environmental stimuli with the administration of chemotherapy (unconditioned stimulus) and its aftereffects (unconditioned response). Support for this view is derived from research demonstrating that patients with ANV are characterized by features that would be predicted from theory and laboratory research to facilitate the acquisition of a conditioned response (e.g., more severe posttreatment nausea/vomiting, higher chemotherapy dose, more emetic drugs) (Redd, 1989). Indeed, Andrykowski and colleagues (1988) found that the occurrence of posttreatment nausea is necessary for the development of ANV.

It has been argued elsewhere (Bovbjerg & Ader, 1986) that the cyclophosphamide-induced conditioned taste aversion and immune suppression in animals is an example of multiple conditioned responses, which are not uncommon when drugs are used as unconditioned stimuli (Wikler, 1973). The cytotoxic drugs used in chemotherapy for cancer have two well-known side effects: nausea and immune suppression. In a manner analogous to the animal studies, chemotherapy patients may thus develop anticipatory immune suppression in addition to anticipatory nausea.

We have recently completed a study designed as a first critical test of the possibility that patients develop anticipatory immune suppression (AIS) in addition to ANV during repeated chemotherapy treatments (Bovbjerg et al., 1990). We hypothesized that measures of immune function would be lower in blood samples obtained in the setting where chemotherapy was about to be administered, as compared to blood samples obtained in the home several days earlier (in the absence of putative conditioned stimuli). This hypothesis was confirmed in a group of women receiving intravenous infusions of chemotherapy in the hospital once every 4 weeks for treatment of ovarian cancer. The possible influences of concurrent nausea and anxiety on immune function were also examined.

Material and methods

Subjects: All participants were women treated for ovarian cancer at Memorial Sloan-Kettering Cancer Center. Eligible patients had: (a) undergone surgical treatment for histologically confirmed Stage III/IV epithelial ovarian carcinoma, (b) no concurrent neoplasms, (c) creatinine clearance over 60 cc per min, (d) normal cardiac status, (e) no clinical hearing deficit, (f) not been treated with chemotherapy for any prior illness, (g) been scheduled to be treated with either five or ten intravenous push infusions of combination chemotherapy, (h) received at least three such infusions, and (i) homes within 2 hr driving time of the laboratory. Subjects ranged in age from 32 to 70 years (M = 51.0; SD = 12.4). In general, patients were capable of performing all activities of daily living (mean Karnofsky Performance rating [14] was 89, SD = 5). Psychosocial adjustment to illness, as assessed by the Global Adjustment to Illness Scale (12), was also high for the group as a whole (M = 97, SD = 8) indicating normal adjustment.Thirty-six consecutive patients were asked to participate. Twenty-seven (75%) agreed and provided informed consent. Seven patients were subsequently dropped from the study: 4 for medical reasons (e.g., change of chemotherapy protocol) and 3 for technical reasons (e.g., had difficult veins for blood collection).

Drug regimen: Patients were scheduled for treatment with intravenous infusions of cyclophosphamide (600 mg/m^2), doxorubicin (40 mg/m^2) and cisplatin (100 mg/m^2) in the hospital every four weeks. Patients were admitted to the hospital the night before chemotherapy and hydrated by intravenous drip with dextrose 5% in water plus half normal saline (175 cc/hr). Sixteen of the 20 patients requested sedation during their hospital stay (prior to the hospital assessment) and received one or more of the following drugs: triazolam (12 patients), pentobarbital (3), alprazolam (2), diazepam (1), promethazine hydrochloride (1), oxycodone hydrochloride (1), hydroxyzine hydrochloride (1), and procholorperazine maleate (1). Chemotherapy was administered by intravenous infusion between 11:00 a.m. and 1:00 p.m. Patients returned home 24-48 hr after completion of the chemotherapy infusion.

Procedure: Patients were entered into the study after they had received at least 3 chemotherapy infusions ($M = 4.1$; $SD = 1.5$). In the 4-week interval before the next chemotherapy treatment, they were telephoned to schedule a home assessment at least 3 days before their forthcoming treatment. To avoid possible circadian effects, home assessments were scheduled for the same time of day as the hospital assessment. During the home assessment an experienced research technician first administered psychological and behavioral questionnaires (see below) requiring approximately 30 minutes. The technician then drew blood samples (40 ml) by venipuncture (to be processed later in the laboratory for assessment of immune function, see below). Three to 8 days later ($M = 4.4$, $SD = 1.6$) patients were assessed in the hospital in the morning, prior to their chemotherapy infusion. Blood samples were collected after the questionnaires were administered.

Psychological and behavioral measures: At the home assessment patients were asked to rate their current level of nausea using visual analog scales (VAS) (Redd et al., 1982). State anxiety was assessed with VAS as well as the Spielberger State-Trait Anxiety Inventory (STAI) (Spielberger et al., 1970). All patients also completed the trait portion of the STAI. At the hospital assessment STAI state ratings of anxiety were collected. Patients were also asked to provide VAS ratings of nausea and anxiety for three points in time: (a) the previous evening; (b) on awakening that morning; and (c) just before chemotherapy. Since the 3 VAS ratings did not differ for either anxiety or nausea in the present study, and previously published findings indicate that such ratings are highly correlated (Andrykowski et al., 1985; Andrykowski et al., 1988), the mean VAS ratings of anxiety and nausea were used in all analyses.

Immune measures: Three aspects of immune function were assessed (cell numbers, proliferative responses to mitogens, and NK cell activity). Uniform immunologic procedures were performed on all blood samples.

Two samples of venous blood were obtained at each assessment: 5 ml was collected in a tube containing EDTA (for Complete Blood Counts [CBC]) and 40 ml was collected in heparinized tubes or syringes (for isolation of peripheral blood mononuclear cells [PBMC]). Automated CBCs were performed by the Hematology Laboratory at Memorial Sloan-Kettering Cancer Center on the day that the blood was collected. PBMC were isolated from heparinized blood by Ficoll-Hypaque density gradient centrifugation as previously described (Bovbjerg et al., 1985). The initiation of the separation procedure was routinely delayed for the blood sample collected in the hospital to approximate the timing for the sample collected in the patient's home (initiated following 1- to 2-hr travel time).

After counting in a hemocytometer, the isolated PBMC were resuspended to 20 x 10^6/ml in media for freezing (50% RPMI-1640 medium and 50% fetal calf serum, [FCS]; Gibco, Grand Island, NY) in an ice bath. The cell suspension was gently mixed with an equal volume of freezing media containing 25% dimethyl sulfoxide (Sigma, St. Louis, MO). Aliquots in freezing vials (Nunc, Denmark) were stored for 1 - 2 days at -70°C and then transferred to a liquid nitrogen freezer. Aliquots of PBMC from each of the two assessments (home and hospital) were later thawed at the same time. To thaw the PBMC, the freezing vials were vigorously shaken in a 37°C water bath. The cells were then washed three times at room temperature in Hank's balanced salt solution (HBSS) (Gibco). Cells were counted and viability was determined by trypan blue exclusion. Cell recovery was routinely greater than 80% and more than 90% of recovered cells were viable.

Proliferative responses to three mitogens were assayed: phytohemagglutinin (PHA; Burrows-Wellcome, Research Triangle Park, NC), concanavalin A (ConA; Sigma), and *Staphyloccus Aureus* Protein A (SPA; Pharmacia, Piscataway, NJ). Single lots of these mitogens were used at optimal concentrations. PBMC were resuspended to 1 x 10^6 viable cells/ml in complete culture medium (CCM) (RPMI-1640 containing 100 units/ml of penicillin, 100 mcg/ml streptomycin, 2 mM glutamine, and 10% heat inactivated pooled human type AB serum) and co-cultured in with an equal volume (100 ul) of: (a) CCM, (b) 4 mcg/ml PHA, (c) 100 mcg/ml ConA, or (d) 80 mcg/ml SPA in triplicate wells of 96-well round-bottomed microculture plates (Corning, Corning, NY). Replicate plates were maintained at 37°C in a humidified atmosphere containing 5% CO_2 for two, four, and six days. Eight hours before the end of the culture period, 1 uCi of tritiated thymidine (^{3}H-Tdr; New England Nuclear, Boston, MA) was added to each well. Cellular proliferation was stopped by freezing the plates (-20°C). Plates were later thawed and cells harvested with an automated cell harvester (Skatron, Sterling, VA) onto glass microfibre sheets (Whatman, Clifton, NJ). The filter disks carrying the incorporated ^{3}H-Tdr were placed in glass vials with 3 ml of scintillation fluid (Liquiscint, National Diagnostics, Parsippany, NJ). Radioactivity was quantified using a Beckman scintillation counter. The results were expressed as the mean counts per minute (cpm) of the triplicate culture wells, unless one of the wells was more than 3 SD different from the mean of the closer two, in which case the mean of two wells was recorded. The proliferative response to mitogen challenge (in cpm) was quantified by subtracting the mean cpm of control triplicates (without mitogen) from the mean cpm of stimulated triplicates. The culture period with maximal response was reported as hospital and home responses did not have different kinetics.

NK cell activity was assayed by chromium release using the highly sensitive K562 erythroleukemic cell line as target (Pross & Maroun, 1984). Cells to be used as targets were washed 3 times in RPMI-1640 at room temperature and resuspended to 1 x 10^7 cells/ml in CCM. They were then cultured with 100 uCi (adjusted for specific activity) of ^{51}Cr (sodium chromate; New England Nuclear) per 10^6 cells for 1 hr at 37°C in a humid atmosphere containing 5% CO_2. Following 3 washes in RPMI-1640 the labeled cells were counted in trypan blue and resuspended to 5 x 10^4 viable cells/ml in CCM. PBMC in CCM were resuspended in aliquots of 3 different concentrations (to provide effector to target ratios of 100:1, 30:1, and 10:1) and 100 ul of each was plated in triplicate in V-bottomed 96-well microtitration plates (Flow Laboratories, McLean, VA) to which 100 ul of the target cells (5 x 10^3) were added. Control wells contained target cells plus 100 ul CCM. The plate was centrifuged gently (80g) for 5 min and then incubated at 37°C in 5% CO_2 for 4 hr. The plate was then centrifuged at 200g for 10 min. Supernatant (100 ul) was removed from each well and transferred to 5 ml plastic tubes (Sarstedt, Princeton, NJ). Radioactivity was counted in a gamma counter (Gamma Trac 1191). Spontaneous release was quantified by the cpm of supernatant from triplicates cultured with CCM, while maximum release was quantified by the cpm of supernatant of such cultures following 3 cycles of freeze-thawing in an acetone/dry ice bath and 37°C water bath. The percentage of specific lysis was calculated as follows:

$$\frac{\text{cpm experimental sample} - \text{cpm spontaneous release}}{\text{cpm maximum release} - \text{cpm spontaneous release}} \times 100$$

Lymphocyte phenotypes present in the PBMC samples were determined by indirect immunofluorescence staining, as previously described by Hillman et al. (1987). Antibodies were either purchased (Ortho Diagnostics, Raritan, NJ) or produced by characterized hybridomas (American Type Culture Collection, Rockville, MD) maintained in the laboratory.

Results

Immune measures: Three classes of measures were used to assess immune function of cells isolated from blood samples: (a) proliferative responses following mitogenic stimulation with PHA, ConA, or SPA; (b) nonspecific cytotoxic activity (NK cell activity); and (c) alterations in the number of specific cell types present. Results were tested by multivariate and univariate analysis of variance (MANOVA and ANOVA) of individual dependent measures. MANOVA indicated a significant within subject effect (home vs. hospital) (F [5, 14] = 43.27, $p < .001$). Results of subsequent ANOVA tests are shown in Table 1.

Tab. 1: Proliferative responses to mitogens[a].

	Assessment Location	
Mitogens	Home	Hospital
PHA	62.7 ± 24.0[b]	51.1 ± 3.9
ConA	26.7 ± 14.9[c]	21.2 ± 3.6
SPA	33.5 ± 9.4[d]	27.5 ± 8.3

[a] Mean counts per minute ± SEM. [b]$F(1,18) = 9.71, p = .006$. [c]$F(1,18) = 5.71, p = .028$. [d]$F(1,19) = 3.15, p = .092$.

Note. Media control cultures were not different ($F[1,19] = 0.7, p = .41$).

As shown in Table 1, responses to the classic T-cell mitogens PHA and ConA were lower when cells were isolated from blood collected in the hospital (hospital PHA and ConA) compared to PBMC isolated from blood collected in the patients' homes (home PHA and ConA).

There was a trend for NK cell activity to be lower in the hospital (M CML = 16.7, SD = 8.4) that at home ($M = 19.6$, $SD = 10.9$) ($F\ (1, 18) = 3.895, p = .064$) at a ratio of 100:1 effector to target cells. There were no significant differences in number of white blood cells, percentage of lymphocytes, absolute number of lymphocytes, or percentage of CD3+, CD8+, or CD4+ cells.

Since 16 of the 20 patients received some sedative drug(s) (possibly immune suppressive) prior to the hospital assessment, it was of interest to determine if the 4 patients who did not receive any drugs showed AIS. To address this possibility, we conducted a separate MANOVA for the mitogen responses for those 4 patients. These patients showed a significant reduction in mitogen response in the hospital compared to the home ($F[5,15] = 12.141, p < 0.001$).

Nausea and anxiety measures: Nausea and anxiety measures were significantly higher in the hospital than in patients' homes (Table 2).

Tab. 2: Nausea and anxiety[a].

Measurement	Assessment Location	
	Home	Hospital
Nausea (VAS)	7.1 ± 2.3[b]	20.4 ± 5.0
Anxiety (VAS)	39.8 ± 5.3[c]	51.2 ± 4.6
Anxiety (STAI)	41.9 ± 2.6[d]	52.2 ± 2.3

[a]Mean ± SEM. [b]$F(1,19) = 14.04, p = .001$. [c]$F(1,19) = 5.12, p = .036$. [d]$F(1,19) = 8.90, p = .008$.

The relationship of psychological and behavioral measures to immune differences: Since patients experienced more anxiety and nausea in the hospital, it was of interest to consider the relationship of these changes to the reduced mitogen responses. Three variables were entered into a hierarchical multiple regression analysis (Cohen & Cohen, 1975) to predict change in mitogen response. As recommended by Cronbach and Ferby (1970), the first predictor variable to be entered was the baseline, the mitogen response at home. We next entered the changes in anxiety levels, and then the change in nausea levels. These three factors accounted for 74% of the variability in ConA differences between home and hospital ($F[3,15] = 6.26, p = .006$), however, 73% of the variability was accounted for by the baseline response alone ($F[1,17] = 43.53, p < .001$). On the other hand, for PHA responses, both the baseline response and changes in nausea made significant contributions to the variability (25% and 30%, respectively), while anxiety did not (Table 3). An identical analysis, using VAS measures of anxiety rather than STAI, yielded similar results.

To examine psychological and behavioral factors that might be related to AIS, patients were divided *post hoc* into those who had lower PHA responses in the hospital ($n = 14$) and those who did not ($n = 5$). These two groups did not differ in trait anxiety (STAI). State anxiety

Tab. 3: Hierarchical multiple regression analysis of change in PHA responses

	Variable		
Measure	Baseline PHA	Change in Anxiety (STAI)	Change in VAS Nausea
Beta	.61	.01	-.56
Multiple R	.50	.50	.74
R^2 Change	.25	.00	.30
F	11.45	.00	10.06
p	.004	.95	.006

$F(3,15) = 15.68$, $p = .0001$.

measures (VAS and STAI) also were not significantly different. However, the pattern of nausea within the subgroups did differ, as indicated by a significant group by time interaction obtained using repeated measures ANOVA ($F[1,17] = 4.736$, $p = .04$). Patients showing AIS had higher levels of nausea in the hospital (hospital vs. home VAS nausea = 23.6 vs. 6.6), while those without AIS did not (hospital vs. home VAS nausea = 5.4 vs. 8.3).

Discussion

Women undergoing repeated infusions of cytotoxic drugs for the treatment of ovarian cancer experienced both decreased immune function and increased nausea when they returned to the hospital for subsequent treatment. Specifically, *in vitro* proliferative responses to the T-cell mitogens, PHA and ConA, were lower for cells isolated from blood collected in the hospital than from blood collected in patients' homes several days earlier (Table 1). Patients also experienced increased nausea and anxiety in the hospital (Table 2). Hierarchical regression analysis (after accounting for baseline responses) indicated that increased anxiety in the hospital did not contribute to the reduced immune function (PHA response), but that increased nausea accounted for 30% of the variance in the reduced PHA response (Table 3). These results merit careful consideration as the observed AIS may well reflect the interaction of psychological, behavioral and biological factors. Moreover, AIS may have clinical relevance to increased risk of infection observed in cancer patients and how cancer treatment is conducted.

Central to the study of both AIS and ANV is the contribution of classical conditioning processes. Was the AIS observed in the present study the result of classical conditioning? It can be argued that, as a consequence of the repeated pairing of hospital stimuli (CS) with immunosuppressive chemotherapy (UCR), patients showed a conditioned immunosuppression response (CR) to the presentation of the CS. Indeed, our findings are consistent with results from experimental conditioning research with laboratory animals (Bovbjeg & Ader, 1986), as well as results from prior investigations of ANV in chemotherapy patients (Redd, 1989). As in research on ANV, our understanding of this phenomenon would be greatly enhanced by experimental studies including the types of control groups used in previous animal experimentation (e.g., noncontingent presentation of CS and US). However, ethical considerations limit our ability to conduct such experiments since exposing humans to immunosuppressive cytotoxic drugs for nontherapeutic reasons would jeopardize their health. Thus, at the present time, conclusions can only be based on the "natural" experiment in which chemotherapy patients are exposed to environmental contingencies that are directly analogous to the classical conditioning paradigm.

Another consideration is the possibility that increased anxiety experienced in the hospital contributes to the observed AIS. Previous research has indicated that people undergoing stressful life events (e.g., medical school examinations) have reductions in various measures of immune function, including mitogen responses and NK cell activity (Kiecolt-Glaser & Glaser, 1988). Since chemotherapy infusions represent life stressors (Nerenz et al., 1982), it is conceivable that the observed AIS was the result of immunosuppressive effects of anxiety. We addressed this possibility with hierarchical multiple regression analyses to quantify the contribution of changes in anxiety (as measured by VAS or STAI) to the reduced PHA response in the hospital. The hypothesis that AIS is the result of increased anxiety was not supported by the results for PHA responses. Similar analysis of the ConA response provided little information about the contribution of anxiety and nausea, since baseline ConA responses accounted for virtually all of the variance in those responses. It should be noted that this finding does not necessarily contradict the notion that anxiety can influence immune function. Rather, changes in patients' anxiety may not have been large enough to induce immune suppression, perhaps because of the relatively high levels of anxiety already evident at the home assessment.

The relationship between anticipatory nausea and AIS must also be considered. One possible explanation for the relationship is that nausea itself may be immunosuppressive. Unfortunately, to our knowledge, no research has explored the impact of nausea on immune function. A more viable explanation for the relationship between nausea and AIS is that simultaneous classical conditioning processes occurred (Redd & Bovbjerg, in prep.). That is, both the emetic and immunosuppressive side effects of chemotherapy were conditioned concurrently. Such multiple conditioned responses are common when drugs are used as unconditioned stimuli (Wikler, 1973). Animals conditioned with cyclophosphamide show both taste aversion and conditioned immune suppression (Bovbjerg & Ader, 1986). What is more, since ANV is thought to be a conditioned response (Morrow & Dobkin, 1989), the finding that increased nausea in the hospital accounted for 30% of the variance in the reduced PHA response is consistent with the concurrent conditioning explanation of AIS.

A number of other factors could contribute to AIS. We considered the possibility that sedative drugs administered to patients in the hospital, to relieve anxiety and facilitate sleep, could be responsible for the observed AIS. However, this possibility is highly unlikely since AIS was observed even in patients who had received no sedative drugs. It is also possible that the biological recovery process following the previous chemotherapy infusion may contribute to the observed AIS. There have been occasional reports that immune recovery from cyclophosphamide follows a biphasic course, with suppression followed by a "rebound overshoot" before a return to baseline (Berd et al., 1984). However, it is difficult to reconcile the notion that AIS is simply the result of the pattern of biologic recovery with our finding that AIS is related to anticipatory nausea. Another possibility is that the observed AIS in part reflects immunosuppressive effects of changes in patients' behavior (e.g., sleep, alcohol consumption) between the home and hospital immune assessments. Although previous human psychoimmune research has not found a significant impact of such changes in behavior on immune suppression associated with stressful events (Kiecolt-Glaser & Glaser, 1988), future studies of AIS should explicitly examine the contribution of behavior changes. Exploration of the mechanisms underlying AIS will be relevant to the overall understanding of how psychological, behavioral, and biological processes interact to modulate immune function.

Regardless of the mechanisms responsible, it is important to consider the potential influence of AIS on the health of the patient receiving chemotherapy. Of particular interest is the contribution of AIS to immune compromise responsible for the high risk of infection in these patients (Bodey, 1986). The impact of AIS on the risk of infection has yet to be determined. Mitogen responses in the hospital, while lower than in patients' homes, remained within normal ranges (Melbye et al., 1986) and were not accompanied by changes in numbers of cells. However, patients who are particularly susceptible to AIS (one patient in the present study had a 50% reduction in PHA response) may indeed have increased risks of infection. For such patients it will be particularly important to develop methods of chemotherapy administration to minimize the opportunity for the development of AIS and to develop intervention techniques to control AIS.

Author notes: Preparation of this article was supported in part by the American Cancer Society, the National Institute of Mental Health, the Bristol Myers Foundation, the Institute for Noetic Sciences, and the Medical Illness Counseling Center. Correspondence should be addressed to Dr. Dana Bovbjerg, Psychoneuroimmunology Laboratory, Box 457, Memorial Sloan-Kettering Cancer Center, New York, NY 10021, U.S.A..We gratefully acknowledge Paul Jacobsen, Bruce Rapkin, Sharon Manne, and Fred Garbrecht for their suggestions on earlier drafts of this article, and Nancy R. Anton for excellent editorial assistance.

References

Ader, R. & Cohen, N. (1991). The influence of conditioning on immune responses. In: Ader, R., Felton, D.L. & Cohen, N. (Eds.). *Psychoneuroimmunology II*. Academic Press, New York.

Andrykowski, M.A., Redd, W.H. & Hatfield, A. (1985). The development of anticipatory nausea: A prospective analysis. *J. Consult. Clin. Psychol.* 53:447.

Andrykowski, M.A., Jacobsen, P.B., Marks, E., Gorfinkle, K., Hakes, T.B., Kaufman, R.J., Currie, V.E., Holland, J.C. & Redd, W.H. (1988). Prevalence, predictors and course of anticipatory measure in women receiving adjuvant chemotherapy for breast cancer. *Cancer* 62:2607.

Berd, D., Maguire, H.C. & Mastrangelo, M.J. (1984). Impairment of concanavalin A-inducible suppressor activity following administration of cyclophosphamide to patients with advanced cancer. *Cancer Res.* 44:1275.

Bodey, G.P. (1986). Infection in Cancer Patients. *Amer. J. Med.* 81:11.

Bovbjerg, D. & Ader, R. (1986). The central nervous system and learning: Feedforward regulation of immune responses. In: Berczi, I. (Ed.) *Pituitary function and immunity*. CRC Press, Boca Raton, FL, p. 252.

Bovbjerg, D.H., Redd, W.H., Maier, L.A., Holland, J.C., Lesko, L.M., Niedzwiecki, D., Rubin, S.C. & Hakes, T.B. (1990). Anticipatory immune suppression and nausea in women receiving cyclic chemotherapy for ovarian cancer. *J. Consult. Clin. Psychol.* 58:153.

Bovbjerg, D., Wang, V., Schwab, R., Lebenger, K., Siskind, G. & Weksler, M. (1985). Lymphocyte transformation induced by autologous cells: XVII. Lower autologous mixed lymphocyte reaction in subjects with a history of hay fever. *Internatl. Arch. Allergy Appl. Immunol.* 78:332.

Carey, M.P. & Burish, T.G. (1989). Etiology and treatment of the psychological side effects associated with cancer chemotherapy: A critical review and discussion. *Psychol. Bull.* 104:307.

Cohen, J. & Cohen, P. (1975). *Applied multiple regression/correlation analysis for the behavioral sciences.* Lawrence Earlbaum, Hillsdale, NJ.

Cronbach, L.J. & Ferby, L. (1970). How we should measure "change" - or should we? *Psychol. Bull.* 74:68.

Derogatis, L.R. (1975). *Global adjustment to illness scale*. Clinical Psychometric Research, Baltimore.

Hillman, J., Russo, C., Weksler, M. & Siskind, G.W. (1987). Evidence for an activated subpopulation of T8-bearing cells in male homosexuals with lymphadenopathy. *Internatl. Arch. Allergy Appl. Immunol.* 84:18.

Karnofsky, D.A. & Burchenal, J.H. (1949). The clinical evaluation of chemotherapeutic agents In: Maclead, C.M. (Ed.) *Evaluation of chemotherapeutic agents* (pp. 199-205). Columbia University Press, New York.

Kiecolt-Glaser, J.K. & Glaser, R. (1988). Psychological influences on immunity: Implications for AIDS. *Amer. Psychologist* 43: 892.

Melbye, M., Biggar, R.J., Ebbesen, P., Neuland, C., Goedert, J.J., Faber, V., Lorenzen, I., Skinhoj, P., Gallo, R.C. & Blattner, W.A. (1986). Long-term seropositivity for human T-lymphotropic virus Type III in homosexual men without the acquired immunodefficiency syndrom: Development of immunological and clinical abnormalities. *Ann. Int. Med.* 104:496.

Morrow, G.R. & Dobkin, P.L. (1989). Anticipatory nausea and vomiting in cancer patients undergoing chemotherapy treatment: Prevalence, etiology and behavioral interventions. *Clin. Psychol. Review* 8:517.

Nerenz, D.R., Leventhal, H. & Love, R.R. (1982). Factors contributing to emotional stress during cancer chemotherapy. *Cancer* 50:1020.

Pross, H.F. & Maroun, J.A. (1984). The standardisation of NK cell assays for use in studies of biological respiratory modifiers. *J. Immunol. Methods* 68:235.

Redd, W.H. (1989). Anticipatory nausea and vomiting and their management. In: Holland, J. & Rowland, J. (Eds.) *Psychooncology*. Oxford University Press, New York (pp. 423-433).

Redd, W.H. & Bovbjerg, D.H. (manuscript in preparation).

Redd, W.H., Andresen, G.V. & Minagawa, R. (1982). Hypnotic control of anticipatory nausea in patients undergoing cancer chemotherapy. *J. Consult. Clin. Psychol.* 50:12.

Spielberger, C.D., Gorsuch, R.I. & Lushene, R.E. (1970). *Test manual for state-trait anxiety inventory*. Consulting Psychologist Press, Palo Alto, CA.

Wikler, A. (1973). Conditioning of successiv adaptive responses to the initial effects of drugs. *Conditional reflex* 8:193.

Chapter 19

Methionine Enkephalin: Activation of Cytotoxic Cells in Cancer and AIDS Patients

Nicholas P. Plotnikoff
Joseph Wybran

University of Illinois, Chicago U.S.A.

Hospital Erasme
Free University of Bruxelles, Belgium

Methionine enkephalin (MEK) has been shown to be derived from T-helper cells (Zurawski et al., 1986). MEK may, therefore, be considered to be a T-cell-derived lymphokine as are interleukin 2 and gamma interferon (Miyajima et al., 1988). Most interestingly, MEK has been shown to increase the number of interleukin 2 receptors as well as levels of interleukin 2 (Wybram et al., 1987). At the same time MEK has also been shown to increase levels of interleukin 1 and gamma interferon (Brown & Van Epps, 1985; Youkilis et al., 1985). These multiple effects of MEK result in activation of macrophages as well as natural killer (NK), killer (K), and lymphokine activated killer (LAK) cells, which are known to destroy tumor cells as well as virus infected cells (Foris et al., 1984; Plotnikoff et al., 1988; Wybran & Plotnikoff, 1989).

The following clinical studies in normal volunteers, cancer and AIDS patients illustrate the multiple actions of MEK.

Normal volunteers

MEK was administered to fourteen normal volunteers at intravenous doses of 1, 10, 50, 100, 150, 200, and 250 μg/kg (Plotnikoff et al., 1987). An example of the immunological findings in a volunteer receiving 150 μg/kg is illustrated in Table 1. The absolute increase of lymphocytes at the end of the 2 and 24 hr periods was due to the increase in B-lymphocytes, T-lymphocytes and NK- cells. At 2 hrs, the B-cells had increased by 72%, the T-lymphocytes by

Tab. 1: Normal volunteer - 150 μg/kg i.v.

	0 hr	2 hr	24 hr
Lymphocytes	21% 1365/mm^3	25% 1600/mm^3	27% 1809/mm^3
B-lymphocytes	13% 177/mm^3	19% 304/mm^3	16% 289/mm^3
T-lymphocytes (E rosettes)	64% 874/mm^3	63% 1008/mm^3	56% 1013/mm^3
Active T-lymphocytes	18% 246/mm^3	40% 640/mm^3	37% 669/mm^3
T -lymphocytes (OKT 11)	74% 1010/mm^3	72% 1152/mm^3	87% 1574/mm^3
T-helper lymphocytes (OKT 4)	33% 450/mm^3	48% 768/mm^3	51% 923/mm^3
T-suppressor lymphocytes (OKT 8)	22% 300/mm^3	20% 320/mm^3	24% 434/mm^3
T-helper/T-suppressor ratio	1.5	2.4	2.1
NK-cells (LEU 7)	13% 177/mm^3	20% 320/mm^3	16% 289/mm
Blastogenesis			
Phytohemagglutinin	571x	950x	609x
Concanavalin A	261x	437x	457x
Pokeweed	69x	112x	93x
Staph A	30x	47x	34x

15% and the NK-cells by 80%. The T-helper cells had increased significantly by the end of the 2 hr period (71%) and continued to increase through the 24 hr period (105%). The T-suppressor cells demonstrated a significant increase at 24 hrs (45%). These two observations were confirmed by the T-helper to T-suppressor ratio which was 2.4 at 2 hrs and 2.1 at 24 hrs. The active T-lymphocytes were significantly elevated at 2 hrs (160%), an increase which persisted at 24 hrs (172%).

The function of the lymphocytes, as evaluated by mitogen-stimulated blastogenesis, was also increased by MEK. PHA, a T-helper cell mitogen, showed a significant increase. ConA, a T-helper and T-suppressor cell mitogen, also resulted in a significant increase in blastogenesis as well as pokeweek, a T-dependent B-cell mitogen, and staph A, a B-cell mitogen.

Cancer patient

In vitro studies with MEK showed that NK cell activity against the target cells (K562) was increased in many cancer patients (lymphoma, leukemia, thyroid, ovarian, gastric, lung, and breast cancer) (Faith et al., 1987). *In vivo* clinical studies were also conducted in several advanced cancer patients with lung cancer, hypernephroma, and melanoma (Plotnikoff et al., 1987). The immunological effects of MEK in a lung cancer patient are shown in Table 2. Significant increases in numbers of cells were seen with lymphocytes, active T-cells, OKT 3, OKT 4, and OKT 8. In terms of blastogenesis, increases were seen with PHA and staph A. Most interesting were the increases seen with interleukin 2 receptor numbers.

AIDS Patients (12)

Kaposi sarcoma patient: This patient was administered MEK at a dose of 25 μg/kg i.v. three times a week. Increases in lymphocytes, OKT 3, OKT 11, OKT 4, and OKT 8 were observed over a time period of 136 days, accompanied by reductions in nodule size and coloration.

Asymptomatic HIV+ patients (13): Increases in cytotoxic T-cells (CD16 and LEU 19) were observed in this patient receiving MEK treatment (60 μg/kg once a week) for four months (Table 4). All immunological measurements were taken seven days after infusion, representing the nadir.

Tab. 2: The immunological effects of MEK in a lung cancer patient (25 μg/kg 3x week).

	Day 1	Day 8	Day 29
Active T-cells	52% 707/mm^3	58% 1183/mm^3	40% 732/mm^3
T-lymphocytes (OKT 3)	64% 870/mm^3	47% 959/mm^3	67% 985/mm^3
T-lymphocytes (OKT 11)	77% 1047/mm^3	50% 1020/mm^3	74% 1088/mm^3
T-helper cells (OKT 4)	36% 489/mm^3	28% 571/mm^3	44% 647/mm^3
T-suppressor cells (OKT 8)	20% 272/mm^3	17% 347/mm^3	22% 323/mm^3
Ratio	1.80	1.65	2.00
Blastogenesis			
Phytohemagglutinin	723x	432x	864x
Concanavalin A	704x	576x	711x
Pokeweed	83x	78x	23x
Staph A	21x	84x	44x
Interleukin-2 receptor	52%	60%	80%
Lymphocytes	1360/mm^3	2040/mm^3	1830/mm^2

Discussion

MEK is derived from the prohormone, proenkephalin A, found in T-helper cells (Zurawski et al., 1986). The release of MEK into the surrounding media results in the activation of NK-K LAK cells (Wybran et al., 1987; Plotnikoff et al., 1988). Thus, MEK may be considered to be a lymphokine as are interleukin 2 and gamma interferon. Since both cancer and AIDS patients have been reported to have deficiencies in lymphokines, reduced cytotoxicity has been observed (Mertlesmann & Welte, 1985; Murray et al., 1984). Consequently, it is not unexpected that immunotherapy has beneficial effects in cancer and AIDS patients (Rosenberg et al., 1988;

Tab. 3: Kaposi sarcoma patient (25 μg/kg 3x week).

	Day 1	Day 2
WBC	5700/mm^3	6100/mm^3
Lymphocytes	1425/mm^3	2074/mm^3
Active T-cells	62% 884/mm^3	
OKT 3	66% 941/mm^3	74% 1535/mm^3
OKT 11	77% 1097/mm^3	73% 1514/mm^3
OKT 4	7% 100/mm^3	8% 165/mm^3
OKT 8	52% 741/mm^3	59% 1224/mm^3
Ratio	0.14	0.14

Tab. 4: Asymptomatic HIV+ patient.

	August 13	October 27
Lymphocytes	19% 1254/mm^3	15% 1012/mm^3
OKT 3	76% 953/mm^3	78% 789/mm^3
OKT 11	85% 1066/mm^3	89% 901/mm^3
OKT 4	24% 301/mm^3	22% 223/mm^3
OKT 8	57% 715/mm^3	55% 557/mm^3
Ratio	0.421	0.400
LEU 11	18% 226/mm^3	36% 364/mm^3
LEU 19	6% 75/mm^3	10% 101/mm^3

Plotnikoff & Miller, 1988). However, the use of interleukin 2 has been accompanied by major side effects (Rosenberg et al., 1988).

In sharp contrast, MEK to date notably lacks major side effects (Plotnikoff et al., 1988). Only minor transient "gut cramps" and facial flushing have been reported. Therefore, it is encouraging to see that MEK can activate cytotoxic cells in cancer and AIDS patients. Perhaps the increased cytotoxicity may reduce metastasis in cancer patients and HIV levels in AIDS patients. Experimental studies in leukemia and melanoma B16 would support such an approach (Plotnikoff & Miller, 1983; Murgo, 1985). More recently, MEK was found to reduce p 24 in AIDS patients (Plotnikoff et al., 1989). We anticipate expanding these clinical studies both in cancer and AIDS patients (Plotnikoff et al., 1986).

References

Bartlett, J.A., Blankenship, K.D., Greenberg, M. et al. (1989). The safety of zidovudine and interleukin-2 in asymptomatic HIV infected patients. *V Int. Conf. AIDS,* Montreal.

Brown, S.L. & Van Epps, D.E. (1985). Beta endorphin, met-enkephalin, and corticotrophin modulate the production of gamma interferon in vitro. *Fed. Proc.* 44, 4:949.

Faith, R.E., Liang, J.H., Plotnikoff, N.P. et al. (1987). Neuroimmunomodulation with enkephalins: In vitro enhancement of natural killer cell activity in peripheral blood lymphocytes from cancer patients. *Nat. Immun. Cell Growth Regul.* 6:88-98.

Foris, G., Medgyesi, G.A., Gyimesi, E. & Hauck, M. (1984). Met-enkephalin induced alterations of macrophage functions. *Mol. Immunol.* 21:747-750.

Mertlesmann, R. & Welte, K. (1985). Restorative immunotherapy with interleukin 2. In: Reif, A.E. & Mitchell, M.S. (Eds). *Immunity to cancer.* Academic, N.Y. pp. 485:498.

Miyajima, A., Miyatake, S., Schreurs, J. et al. (1988). Coordinate regulation of immune and inflammatory responses by T-cell derived lymphokines. *FASEB J.* 2, 9 :2462-2473.

Murgo, A.J. (1985). Inhibition of B16-BL6 melanoma growth in mice by methionine-enkephalin. *JNCI 75,* 2:341-344.

Murray, H.W., Rubin, B.Y., Masur, H. & Roberts, R.B. (1984). Impaired production of lymphokines and immune (gamma) interferon in the acquired immunodeficiency syndrome. *N.E.J.M.* 310:883-889.

Plotnikoff, N.P. & Miller, G.C. (1983). Enkephalins as immunomodulators. *Int. J. Immunopharm.* 5:437-441.

Plotnikoff, N.P., Faith, R.E., Murgo, A.J. & Good, R.A. (1986). *Enkephalins-endorphins: Stress and the immune system.* Plenum, N.Y..

Plotnikoff, N.P., Miller, G.C., Nimeh, N. et al. (1987). Enkephalins and T-cell enhancement in normal volunteers and cancer patients. *Ann. N.Y. Acad. Sci.* 496:608-619.

Plotnikoff, N.P., Miller, G.C., Nimeh, N.F. & Wybran, J. (1987). Methionine enkephalin: immunomodulator in normal volunteers, cancer and AIDS patients. *Mem. Inst. Oswaldo Cruz, Rio de Janeiro 82*, S11: 67-73.

Plotnikoff, N.P., Miller, G.C. & Wybran, J. (1987). *ACTH and endorphins in hormones and immunity.* Berczi, I., Kovacs, (eds) MTP Press, Norwell, MA pp.130-144.

Plotnikoff, N.P., Miller, G.C., Mineh, N. & Wybran, J. (1988). Methionine enkephalin: Enhancement of cytotoxic T-cells in ARC patients. *IV Int. Conf. AIDS, Stockholm,* June 1988.

Plotnikoff, N.P., Miller, G.C. & Wybran, J. (1989). Activation by methionine enkephalin: Enhancement of cytotoxic T-cells in HIV+ patients. *V Int. Conf. AIDS, Montreal,* p. 400.

Rosenberg, S.A., Lotze, M.T. & Mule, J.J. (1988). New approaches to the immunotherapy of cancer using interleukin-2. *Ann. Int. Med.* 108:853-865.

Wybran, J. & Plotnikoff, N.P. (1989). Enhancement of immunological mechanisms, including LAK induction by methionine enkephalin. *7th Int. Cong. Immun. Berlin.*

Wybran, J., Schandene, L., van Cooren, J.P. et al. (1987). Immunologic properties of methionine-enkephalin, and therapeutic implications in AIDS, ARC and Cancer. *Ann. N.Y. Acad. Sci.* 496:108-114.

Youkilis, E., Chapman, J., Woods, E. & Plotnikoff, N.P. (1985). In vivo immunostimulation and increased in vitro production of interleukin I (IL-1) activity by met-enkephalin. *Int. J. Immunopharm.* 7, 3:79.

Zurawski, G., Benedik, M., Kamb, B.J. et al. (1986). Activation of T-helper cells induces abundant preproenkephalin in RNA synthesis. *Science* 323:772.

Chapter 20

Breast Cancer - Is there a Psychological Risk Factor in Disease Progression?

Maggie Watson

The Royal Mardsen Hospital
and Institute of Cancer Research, U.K.

An area which is hotly debated concerns the issue of whether psychological factors can play a role in either carcinogenesis or cancer progression. Renewed interest in the relationship between psychological factors and cancer stems from recent evidence that immune responses are conditionable. Rapid advances in the area of immunology, over the last twenty years, have allowed a better understanding of the relationship of cellular activity to endocrine and nervous system responses. In order to establish a psychosomatic model of cancer, there are a number of important basic requirements. Firstly, it would be necessary to identify particular psychological responses and confirm their more frequent occurrence in those who develop cancer. Secondly, these responses would need to be associated with physical changes considered to contribute to the promotion of cancer. Research findings obtained by the King's College Hospital and Royal Marsden Hospital Research Groups are presented in relation to these issues.

Back in the early 1970's, the model we followed was very much influenced by Burnet's (1970) theory of immunosurveillance (see Fig.).

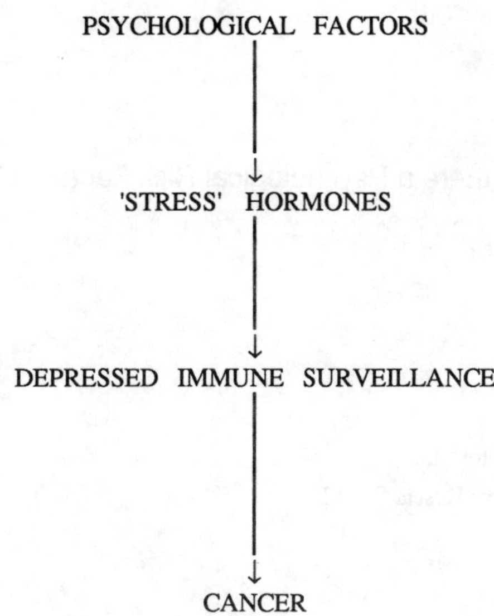

This involved the idea that psychological factors would serve to affect the release of stress hormones which in turn acted upon immune responses with the body's immune surveillance system being somehow depressed (Pettingale, 1985). According to this model, the immunodepression would act to increase the risk of breast cancer. In following this model through, our research group embarked upon a series of studies, and one of the earliest observations was that women with breast cancer were more likely to control feelings of anger than an age-matched group with benign breast disease (Morris et al., 1981). Since then, we have replicated this finding using a newly developed measure of emotional control and confirmed that women with breast cancer are significantly more likely to suppress anger than those with benign breast disease and a normal matched control group (Watson et al., 1985). Subsequent studies undertaken using the same measures in Italy (Grassi et al., 1985; Grassi et al., 1986) and Greece (Anagostopoulos & Vassilaros, 1986) have confirmed this finding. A recent review (Gross, 1989) of psychological responses in cancer patients has also shown that there are at least 18 separate studies where emotional control is implicated as a factor influencing cancer prognosis.

Although control of anger appears to be central, a number of related attributes have been identified. We also found that breast cancer patients reported a tendency toward social compliance and unassertiveness (Watson et al., 1985), and it was observed that this might constitute a behavioural style which we have since labelled Type "C" (Morris, 1980; Greer & Watson, 1985).

More recent work has suggested that the Type "C" behaviour is the polar opposite to the Type "A" behaviour associated with increased risk of heart disease. However, much of this research rests heavily upon questionnaire data, and some validation of this phenomenon was important. In one study, behaviour was assessed under controlled conditions in order to discover if patients actually behaved as they reported. Patients were presented with emotionally challenging stimuli and their responses were observed. The data indicated that women with breast cancer were less emotionally responsive and, for those with a tendency to adopt a defensive style of coping, there was increased electrodermal activity. From these data we concluded that breast cancer patients showed a tendency to control negative emotional responses and this was reflected in their behaviour. Autonomic responses did not differ between breast cancer patients and controls, but for those who coped using a "defensive" style there was an associated increase in electrodermal activity.

In following through the original model we have also examined immunological responses under conditions of stress. To do this, we turned away from cancer patients, whose immune system might well be compromised by the disease, and instead examined psychological and immunological responses in a cancer-free sample of bereaved spouses (Pettingale et al., 1989). The results confirmed that high anxiety and pathological grief were associated with a decreased number of natural killer cells. More intriguing, however, given our previous findings was a highly significant association between control of anger and a higher proportion of Helper "T" cells in peripheral blood samples and an overall correlation between emotional control and a *decreased* number of NK cells. There were two conclusions from this study: first, that control of anger was significantly associated with more psychiatric symptoms and, second, that the data supported the concept of neuro-endocrine modulation of the immune system. However, these data did not suggest that the overall effect was immunosuppressive or that there were any immunological changes of *clinical* significance. It seems likely that, if stress or psychological responses have any physical concomitants, then their most significant influence may be through the neuro-endocrine system and this deserves to be researched further.

In a previous study (Greer et al., 1979) we had observed that certain psychological responses were related to prognosis among women with breast cancer. This study indicated that breast cancer patients showing a helpless or stoical attitude towards their disease, when measured three months after breast surgery, were more likely to be dead at ten- and thirteen-year (Pettingale et al., 1985) follow-up than those who had initially shown a "fighting spirit". In this original study patients were allocated to one of the psychological categories according to their responses in a clinical interview. This had certain drawbacks. It was necessary to be trained in the interview technique and also the patient was allocated to only one of the categories whereas, in practice, coping may be more complex than this original method allowed. Since then we have developed a questionnaire measure of assessing psychological responses (Watson et al., 1988), and this is presently being used in a new study measuring psychological responses among a number of patients with mixed cancer diagnoses as well as breast cancer. In our previous studies no clear association was found between the psychological responses described (see Table 1) and emotional control. Data drawn from our most recent study (Watson et al., 1989), however, indicate a clear association between control of anger and the tendency to adopt either a fatalistic or helpless response to the diagnosis of breast cancer:

Fighting Spirit (FS) Fully accepts the diagnosis, uses the word 'cancer', is determined to fight the illness, tries to obtain as much information as possible about it and adopts an optimistic attitude; may see the illness as a challenge.

Helplessness/Hopelessness (H) Is engulfed by knowledge of the diagnosis, finds it difficult to think of anything else, daily life is considerably disrupted by fears concerning cancer and, possibly, death: adopts a wholly pessimistic attitude.

Anxious Preoccupation (AP) Reacts to the diagnosis with marked persistent anxiety ± accompanying depression, actively seeks information about cancer but tends to interpret this pessimistically; worries that aches and pains indicate spread or recurrence of cancer, may seek 'cures' from various sources including so-called alternative treatments.

Fatalism (stoic acceptance) (F) Accepts the diagnosis, does not seek further information, adopts a fatalistic attitude.

Avoidance (Denial) (A) Refuses to accept the diagnosis of cancer or avoids using the word 'cancer', or admits the diagnosis but denies or minimises the seriousness.

These data are exciting because they suggest a possible link between emotional control, psychological responses we have previously described, and cancer prognosis.

Taking all of our studies together, it would appear that emotional control, particularly control of anger, is related to an increased incidence of psychological morbidity and, in a bereaved sample, to changes in immune responses. Control of anger, in turn, is linked to the tendency to show helpless and fatalistic response when coping with a diagnosis of breast cancer. Perhaps then an assessment of Type "C" behaviour would be useful to make, along with the psychological responses we have previously described.

Despite these interesting findings relating to psychological responses observed among breast cancer patients, we are still a long way from understanding their effects on immune function. Indeed, many studies which have shown immune responses to be conditionable have produced results which were of statistical significance but of no *clinical* significance. Yet more important, perhaps, is the issue of the role of immune responses in cancer. Apart from AIDS-related tumours, there is some disagreement about whether immune responses play any significant role in cancer. A recent review of this area suggests that our knowledge of the role of immunological factors in the development of breast cancer is extremely limited (Hall, 1988). However, the immune surveillance concept has not been discarded. Instead, it has been suggested that it be broadened to include additional immunological mechanisms and the idea of local specialisation of immune function. Now, for example, new information on oncogenes and their products suggests possible targets for immuno-regulation of certain cancers. At this stage more research is needed on local immune changes and, for breast cancer, on any important influences of neuro-endocrine responses which might link psychological responses to the disease process.

In conclusion, predictions based on a psycho-biological model would be:

i) Type "C" behaviour - particularly emotional suppression - may be a risk factor in the progression of certain cancers.

ii) Under conditions of stress Type "C" individuals will show a specific biological response pattern.

These would be necessary but not sufficient in themselves to constitute increased risk in cancer. At the present time more research is needed to operationalize the Type "C" concept and the introduction of prospective studies will be needed to determine whether it constitutes a risk and what proportion of risk in breast cancer progression.

Acknowledgements

This presentation was based on work undertaken by members of the Faith Courtauld Unit and the Cancer Research Campaign Psychological Medicine Group. Co-workers were: Steven Greer, Tina Morris, Keith Pettingale and Dudley Tee. Many other people have assisted with some part of the studies cited, and their help is gratefully acknowledged.The author is presently a research fellow supported by the Cancer Research Campaign.

References

Anagostopoulos, F. & Vassilaros, S.T. (1986). Personality attributes of women who develop breast cancer. Paper presented at the *16th European Conference on Psychosomatic Research*, Athens, Greece.

Burnet, F.M. (1970). The concept of immunological surveillance. *Prog. Exp. Tumor. Res.* 13:1-27.

Grassi, L., Nappi, G., Susa, A. & Molinari, S. (1986). Eventi stressanti, supporto sociale e caratteristiche psicologiche in pazienti affette da carcinoma della mammella. In: Pancheri, P. & Biondi, M. (Eds.) *Lo Stress, le emozioni, il cancro*. Il Pensiero Scientifico, Roma.

Grassi, L., Watson, M. & Greer, S. (1985). Le Courtauld Emotional Control Scale (CECS) di Watson e Greer. *Bollettino di Psicologia Applicata* 176:3-10.

Greer, S., Morris, T. & Pettingale, K.W. (1979). Psychological response to breast cancer: effect on outcome. *Lancet* 2:785-787.

Greer, S. & Watson, M. (1985). Towards a psychobiological model of cancer: psychological considerations. *Soc. Sci. Med.* 20:773-777.

Gross, J. (1989). Emotional expression in cancer onset and progression. *Soc. Sci. Med.*12:1239-1248.

Hall, J. (1988). Immunity and Cancer. In: Tiffany, R. & Pritchard, P. (Eds.). *Oncology for Nurses and Health Care Professionals*. Harper & Row, 125-144.

Morris, T. (1980). A 'Type C' for cancer? Low trait anxiety in the pathogenesis of breast cancer. *Cancer Detect. Prev*. 3:102.

Morris, T., Greer, S., Pettingale, K.W. & Watson, M. (1981). Patterns of expression of anger and their psychological correlates in women with breast cancer. *Journal of Psychosom. Res*. 25:111-117.

Pettingale, K.W. (1985). A review of psychobiological interactions in cancer patients. In: Watson, M. & Morris, T. (Eds.). *Psychological Aspects of Cancer Advances in the Biosciences*. Pergamon Press, Vol. 49.

Pettingale, K.W., Morris, T., Greer, S. & Haybittle, J.L. (1985). Mental attitudes to cancer: an additional prognostic factor. *Lancet* 1:750.

Pettingale, K.W., Watson, M., Tee, D.E.H., Inayat, Q. & Alhag, A. (1989). Pathological grief following conjugal bereavement. *Stress Medicine* 5:77-83.

Watson, M., Greer, S., Young, J., Inayat, Q., Burgess, C. & Robertson, B. (1988). Development of a questionnaire measure of adjustment to cancer. The MAC Scale. *Psychological Medicine* 18:203-209.

Watson, M., Greer, S., et al. (1989). The relationship between emotional control, mental adjustment to cancer and psychological morbidity in a group of recently diagnosed breast cancer patients. In preparation.

Watson, M., Pettingale, K.W. & Greer, S. (1985). Stress reactions and autonomic arousal in breast cancer patients. In: Watson, M. & Morris, T. (Eds.) *Psychological Aspects of Cancer. Advances in the Biosciences*. Pergamon Press, Vol 49.

Index

Authors

Subjects

From the

World Health Organisation, Division of Mental Health

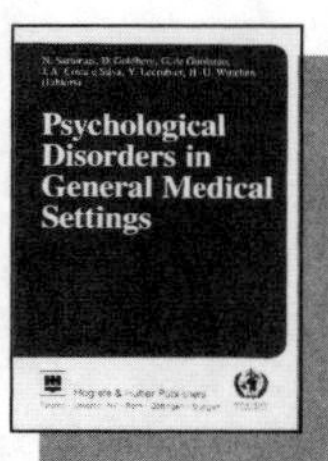

Sartorius/Goldberg/
Costa e Silva/Lecrubier/
de Girolamo/Wittchen (Eds.)

Psychological Disorders in General Medical Settings

Physicians and nurses are constantly presented with patients experiencing an amazing variety of psychological disorders, but these problems are often completely unrecognized, and frequently mistreated.

In this very practical book, the authors examine the magnitude of this problem, discuss the nature, form, and course of the most commonly encountered psychological disorders, and give step-by-step descriptions of helpful diagnostic techniques. Also included is an extensive annotated directory of mental health training courses and manuals that deal with the relationship between those physical and psychological disorders most likely to be of practical interest to a wide variety of clinical health-care professionals.

DM 68.– / US$ 39.– / £ 24.–
ISBN 3-456-81851-3

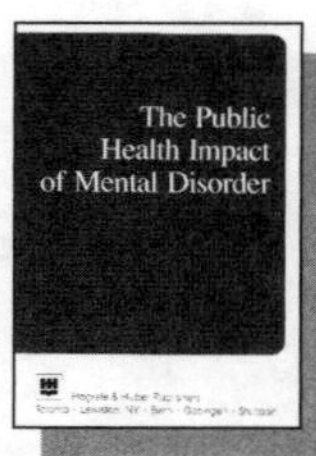

Goldberg/Tantam (Eds.)

The Public Health Impact of Mental Disorder

This volume addresses specific examples of mental health disorders of major public concern such as schizophrenia, depression, AIDS, and suicide, which can be practically and effectively treated through the development of public health policies incorporating the methods of social psychology. The field of social psychiatry has played a pivotal role in putting mental health care into the orbit of public health. The issue now is to define the possibilities and limitations of social psychiatry as a practical tool in aiding the resolution of major social problems.

DM 88.– / US$ 48.– / £ 32.50
ISBN 3-456-81901-3

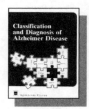

Hovaguimian/Henderson/
Katchatourian/Orley(Eds.)

Classification and Diagnosis of Alzheimer Disease
An International Perspectives

This book provides an interdisciplinary approach to the diagnosis of Alzheimer's Disease considering clinical, psychometric, brain imaging and biological methods. The five main sections are: 1) International Perspectives on Clinical Diagnosis; 2) Standardized Assessment in Diagnosis; 3) Brain Imaging Techniques; 4) Neuropathology; 5) Outlook for the Future.

DM 128.– / US$ 68.– / £ 45.90
ISBN 3-456-81680-4

Sartorius/Regier/Jablensky/Burke/Hirschfeld (Eds.)

Sources and Traditions of Contemporary Psychiatry

This book is a highly readable overview of the origins and the current state of the principles, key concepts, and applications of psychiatry. Special emphasis is given to the various "schools" of the subject and their key philosophical and practical differences. *Contents:*
• The French Psychiatric Tradition • Russian and Soviet Psychiatry • The U.S. Scene • Approaches to Diagnosis and Classification in German-speaking Psychiatry • The Scandinavian School • Spanish Psychiatry

DM 98.– / US$ 49.– / £ 35.40
ISBN 3-456-81821-1

Shepherd/Sartorius (Eds.)

Non-Specific Aspects of Treatment

Recognition is growing in scientific circles that many medical and psychiatric problems cannot be solved through narrowly defined biological approaches. Rather, environmental and psychosocial factors, as well as complex interactions at the psychologic level contribute to the effectiveness of therapeutic intervention.

DM 68.– / US$ 39.– / £ 23.95
ISBN 3-456-81681-2

Hogrefe & Huber Publishers

P.O.Box 51
Lewiston, NY 14092
USA
(716) 282-1610

12 Bruce Park Avenue
Toronto, Ontario
M4P 2S3 CANADA
(416) 482-6339

Verlag Hans Huber

Länggass-Strasse 76
CH-3000 Bern 9
SWITZERLAND
(031) 242533

Verlag Hans Huber GmbH

Robert-Bosch-Breite 25
D-3400 Göttingen
GERMANY
(0551) 50 688-30

Basic Facts in Psychiatry

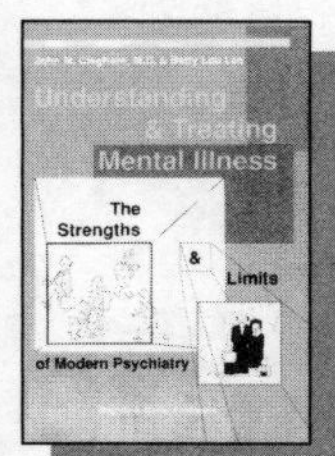

Cleghorn, J.M.; M.D., McMaster University, Hamilton, Ontario, Canada
Lee, B.L., Hamilton, Ontario, Canada

Understanding and Treating Mental Illness
The Strength and Limits of Modern Psychiatry

"This book is a good compendium of current state of our knowledge about the diagnosis, treatment, and options. I think it will do a great deal to enlighten the public about some of the critical and important issues regarding psychiatry and psychiatric care."

Dr. P.J. Fink, Past President, American Psychiatric Association

The book has been especially designed for use by mental health professionals as a teaching device, and for distribution to patients' relatives in connection with an initial consultation, to encourage the family members to see the big picture regarding the various techniques available today.
250 pages, softcover
Fr. 26.– / DM 29.80 / US$ 16.95 / CAN$ 19.95 / £ 10.95
ISBN 3-456-81829-7, ISBN 0-920887-73-2

Jenike, M.A.; M.D., Dept. of Psychiatry, Harvard Medical School, Boston, MA, USA
Asberg, M., Dept. of Psychiatry and Psychology, Karolinska Institute, Stockholm, Sweden (Editors)

Understanding Obsessive-Compulsive Disorder (OCD)

Now that obsessive-compulsive disorder (OCD) can often be successfully treated, it is being increasingly diagnosed and studied. Major advances have been made in our understanding of its causation, symptomatology, and treatment. Most OCD patients are relatively normal people who can be helped to lead completely well adjusted lives, once this disorder is remedied. They usually respond best to a combination of drug treatment with behavioral therapy. This informative report contains practical advice for doctors on the recognition and management of OCD - for the ulimate benefit of their patients.
67 pages, hardcover
Fr. 25.– / DM 29.– / US$ 16.– / CAN$ 19.–
ISBN 3-456-81923-4, ISBN 0-88937-046-X

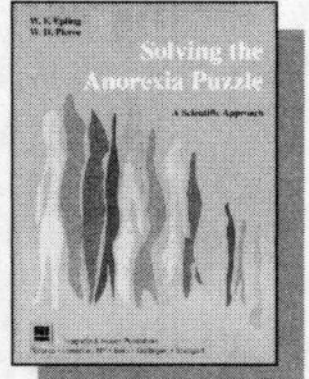

Epling, W.F., Department of Psychology, University of Alberta, Canada
Pierce, W.D., Department of Psychology, University of Alberta, Canada (Editors)
Foreword by Beaumont, P.J.V., Department of Psychiatry, University of Sydney, Australia

Solving the Anorexia Puzzle
A Scientific Approach

This well-organized and highly readable title explains our current knowledge regarding anorexia in general, and activity anorexia in particular, which, the authors argue, any person can develop under certain conditions.
The book first provides an interesting critical review of the diverse medical and psychological perspectives on anorexia nervosa, and contends that many traditional viewpoints on this problem can be misleading: anorexia is often not a mental illness and should, therefore, not be treated as such. In particular, activity anorexia results from a complex interplay of biology, behavior, and culture.
The authors suggest that excessive activity in anorectics is not a secondary symptom, but rather a central feature in understanding the disorder. From the results of laboratory experiments on animals, and from clinical observations of patients, the authors suggest that people in sports, athletics, and fitness programs may develop eating disorders due to the impact of how excessive training can change patterns of food intake. Of course, also methods of treating and preventing anorexia are evaluted in the book.
256 pages, hardcover
Fr. 45.– / DM 50.– / US$ 34.95 / CAN$ 39.95 / £ 18.50
ISBN 3-456-81865-3, ISBN 0-88937-034-6

Hogrefe & Huber Publishers
P.O.Box 51
Lewiston, NY 14092
USA
(716) 282-1610

12 Bruce Park Avenue
Toronto, Ontario
M4P 2S3 CANADA
(416) 482-6339

Verlag Hans Huber
Länggass-Strasse 76
CH-3000 Bern 9
SWITZERLAND
(031) 242533

Verlag Hans Huber GmbH
Robert-Bosch-Breite 25
D-3400 Göttingen
GERMANY
(0551) 50 688-30